AUTOPHAGY FASTING

A Practical Guide on How to Activate Autophagy
Safely

(Discover How to Activate Autophagy Safely
Through Intermittent Fasting)

Robert Buie

Published by Tomas Edwards

*Autophagy Fasting: A Practical Guide on How to Activate
Autophagy Safely (Discover How to Activate Autophagy
Safely Through Intermittent Fasting)*

ISBN 978-1-989744-96-3

Legal & Disclaimer

The information contained in this book is not designed to replace or take the place of any form of medicine or professional medical advice. The information in this book has been provided for educational and entertainment purposes only.

The information contained in this book has been compiled from sources deemed reliable, and it is accurate to the best of the Author's knowledge; however, the Author cannot guarantee its accuracy and validity and cannot be held liable for any errors or omissions. Changes are periodically made to this book. You must consult your doctor or get professional medical advice before using any of the

Table of Contents

Introduction

This book aims to enhance your understanding of autophagy. It gives you relevant information to give you a better appreciation of autophagy and how it helps the body to function optimally.

The book contains concrete strategies about how to induce the condition. It provides concrete and specific instructions on what you can do to promote autophagy.

The book explains how fasting may be the best strategy for inducing autophagy. It outlines the different intermittent fasting strategies. It goes into detail about how to apply the strategies in your daily life.

With detailed instructions at your fingertips, you can choose which strategy works well for your lifestyle. You can even develop your own strategy by combining two or more of the techniques that the book provides.

After reading this book, I hope that you will be able to use what you have learned to achieve your long-term health goals.

Thanks again for downloading this book, I hope you enjoy it!

Chapter 1: the age of gluttony

Without leaving your home and simply turning on the television or watching food related videos on the internet, you are exposed to the desire of having food and lots of it. When you visit fast food restaurants, the servings are large, and many are quite unhealthy they do not contain the macronutrients, that the body needs to maintain optimal health. They are what many people refer to as *"empty calories".*

To get the right amount of nutrients, you need to eat a variety of foods. This is a sensible approach; if you look at it this way, the more you broaden the amount that you eat, the greater the chance for you to get the nutrient that you need. Even if you love peanuts, why not have mixed nuts instead. You will get a boost of Vitamin E from almonds and also a dosage of plant based omega 3 from the walnuts in the mix. Imagine if there were raisins and other dried fruit in the mix if you get a Trail mix pack.

This means that there Will be a greater amount of nutrients to be had. This can also be said if you decide to have a salad. Whether you choose to use lettuce or kale, try to have a mixture of carrots that are rich in vitamin A (your eyes will love it) and also your body will be happy with the tomatoes which are a good source of lycopene.

However, a contradictory scientific advisory has stated that probably, this variety of foods is probably not as good for you as we think. Based on the American Heart Association's publication in the journal entitled *"Circulation"*, variety in your diet may not help you to maintain a healthy weight or even eat healthily.

In fact, even though there are examples of healthy options for variations in our diet shared above, this outline isn't what is being put into practice today. Studies show that even though we are eating a variety of foods, the choices that we make are quite questionable. Today, we are more so consuming highly processed foods that are unhealthy and less of those that are of a healthier choice. So, even if we are following the advice of eating a variety of foods, we still see an increase in obesity and other lifestyle diseases.

This situation is compounded by the fact that so many of us are unable to actually identify when we are full. Even when our stomachs are filled, we still desire to have the dessert at the end of the meal. This actually has to do with the sensor in our body that signals satiety.

Our body is telling us that we need to eat a main Savory meal and then a dessert because according to David Katz, MD, MPH, *"We tend to fill up in a food and flavor specific manner".* Technically, this is eating a variety of foods but those that bring more harm to our bodies than good.

Even though we say we are diversifying the foods that we eat, we mix it with poor food choices. Our meals are normally filled with processed foods, drinks that are loaded with sugars and sweeteners and even those with much refined grains (such as white rice and bleached flours). We consume less of those foods that are unprocessed or minimally processed such as fruits, vegetables and fish.

Coupled with a less active lifestyle, we see ourselves gaining much weight. So, if we are really interested in eating healthily, we should consider to avoid in totality or even lessen our consumption of those oh so tempting donuts, chips, fries and even cheeseburgers. The variety in our meals should not include eating too much of those unhealthy foods too often.

So, what do we eat that will allow us to lose weight and maintain it? This means that we will have to change our current diet and be more knowledgeable about our food choices. Normally when we hear of people going on a diet, we are thinking of boring meals that are repeated over and over. Who really loves monotony in their eating plan? However, there are still some foods that are of poor quality and that are highly processed that we need to avoid.

Foods to avoid

According to the National Institute of Health, many deaths within the United States are related to heart diseases. The data they present states that this disease is responsible for one in four deaths. With such data, it is easy to state that this is the leading cause of death in America.

Even though numerous factors play their part in the development of heart disease (genetics, obesity, smoking, inactivity, etc.), research has shown that our diets do play a great role in our risk of heart disease.

So, if we consume excessively some of the unhealthy foods that we will look at shortly, then we are more likely to suffer from heart disease. Therefore, it is important for us to now know the foods that are damaging to our health, and this will help you to make healthier lifestyle choices.

Fried Foods: Fried chicken and other fried foods have become a staple in our diets. However, we need to note that foods such as these contain a large amount of saturated fat due to the way they are prepared (fried in oil or fat). Saturated fat is actually one of the major contributors to us having high cholesterol and heart disease.

Even though fat is one of the macronutrients that our body needs, the oils that our foods are fired in contain what is known as trans-fats and these are very harmful to our overall health. They contribute to raising our bad cholesterol levels (LDL, low-density) and lowering our good cholesterol (HDL, high-density lipoproteins). These types of fats increase inflammation in our bodies, and this increases the onset of heart disease.

Therefore, it is suggested that we decrease our intake of these types of foods. This means that we can eat the same types of foods when they are prepared in different ways. Better food preparation methods include broiling, baking and grilling. This means that our foods will not come in contact with those unhealthy saturated and trans-fat. So, why not choose grilled or baked chicken instead? Baked potatoes and poached fish are also good items to have on our menus.

Sugar rich foods: Almost every processed food that we eat contains a large quantity of added sugars. We may not see the word ***"sugar"*** on the label, but we will see terms such as corn syrup, dextrose, fructose, glucose, malt syrup, maltose, molasses, and sucrose. These are added for flavor and will drastically increase the calorie content of these foods.

In addition, processed foods have few nutrients and many of the nutrients that we see on the label do not come from natural sources. It is not to say that we should omit sugar completely from our diets. However, if we consume excess amounts, we are also at a greater risk for heart disease.

This is supported by research conducted and published in the February 2012 issue of *"circulation"*. The study states that 42,883 men were observed to note their sugar intake over 22 years. It was found that over the number of participants in the study, 3,683 of them had heart attacks. The conclusion of the study notes that those who consumed a lot of sugar-laden drinks are *"20 percent more likely to suffer from heart attacks"*, than the men who did not.

Therefore, choosing healthy choices such as unprocessed foods (whole foods) is better than consuming a high quantity of sugars in our diet. So, the next time you go grocery shopping or order take out, try to avoid pastries, frostings, candy, sodas and even pancake syrup.

Refined Grains: That pasta that we love to eat with marinara sauce is most likely made from enriched flour. This, along with white rice, is considered to be made from refined grains. When grains have been processed to this extent, they lose much of their nutritional value. It is recommended that we consume more whole grains in our diets.

These are better at helping us to reduce our risk of heart disease. Brown rice or wild rice is better than the more prevalent white rice. Oatmeal and even bran flakes are also better than the sugary cereals we normally see on the shelves in the supermarket.

These foods are rich in fiber and help us to feel full for longer, thus decreasing our calorie intake and help us to properly manage our weights. So, the next time you visit your grocery store, it is wise that you avoid purchasing flour tortillas, white bread, and even your favorite cereals.

Based on our identification of sugar, fried foods and refined grains playing a great role in the increase in obesity and heart disease, below is a list of foods that we need to avoid ore at in limited quantities. These are just to show that processed foods can be very harmful to our health.

Store bought frosting: Frosting, in general, is not recommended because of its high sugar content. But if you wish to indulge a bit, you should avoid the prepackaged ones that are sold in stores.

Placing them on our cakes and other pastry items may be quite tasty, but we should consider that they are loaded with trans fats. We already looked at the harm that these trans fats will do to our bodies.

We need to consider that these fat contributes to high cholesterol levels, lowing the good cholesterol in our bodies which then will lead to inflammation, increase in our girth (belly fat) and placing us at a higher risk of heart disease and diabetes.

Bagels: Bagels are the go-to morning food for many. They are indeed great with cream cheese and many other toppings. Again, this is made of processed grains and will be detrimental to our overall health. But research also shows that based on the high glycemic index that they have there is seen negative effects on out aging and actually helps to increase acne. An English muffin or even whole-grain toast are better options when you wish to break your fast.

Baked products: We are not talking about those that we prepare at our home. We are more likely to know what are in these products and will be better able to make better choices as it relates to what we consume. The culprits here are these convenient treats that we may purchase at stores that are highly processed.

So, those packaged muffins that come in a variety of flavors, these doughnuts and cakes are a no-no Why? We already know that they are high in sugars and are loaded with calories that do not provide much nutritional value to our diet. We should also consider that they are not readily digested, and this is due to the fact that these foods are highly processed.

They are pumped with preservatives (that do us more harm than good) to ensure that they have a longer shelf life. This is the same reason why Twinkies are thought to be one of the foods that will not spoil even if the world experiences an apocalypse. Again, we will see the same negative effect as discussed above if we consume bagels. In addition, we may also feel and look puffy or bloated.

Sodas: We have already stated that this is not something we should consume excessively. These drinks have an excessive amount of sugar, more than what is recommended that we should intake daily. One soda can contain up to 10 packets of sugar which is way more than the recommended 24 grams or six teaspoons that we should limit ourselves to.

Sugar rich cereals: These contain too much sugar. We see on the television daily advertisements that try to lure us to buy these food items that are not good for us. So, even though we love toe at our Frosted Flakes, Fruit Loops, Cheerios and the high sugar and gluten content actually increases inflammation in our bodies. Gluten is also a trigger for an increase in acne breakouts and redness of the skin.

Sugar free options of cereal are very difficult to find but choose those that are low in sugar and gluten. Rex Chex and the plain ole cornflakes are good options. Just be sure the list of ingredients on the boxed to ensure that you are not loading up on sugar.

Stick butter or margarine: Margarine is normally loaded with trans fat and is used in the preparation of many food items that we love to consume. Such as crackers and pastries, even in the ever so loved microwave popcorn. In order to limit our intake of these sources of trans fat, we should check labels as we need to keep our cholesterol levels in check.

Tomato sauce in jars: This is used a lot in fast and easy cooking. They are purchased to make many tomato based recipes such as pizza and spaghetti dishes. Though they are deemed to be savory food items, they are actually sweet as they are loaded with a lot of sugars. It is best that you prepare your own tomato sauce at home.

Bacon: We noted that food eaten in excess is not necessarily good for you. We consume bacon with our breakfast, as salad toppings and even on our sandwiches. We need to be careful as a strip of bacon has up to 45 calories and is high in fat and sodium. We shouldn't forget that it has high quantities of sodium nitrate as this helps to preserve the meat. So, do note that this food shouldn't be eaten in excess.

Maraschino cherries: This is a tasty topping to add to our sundaes and cocktails. This is preserved in a jar and had a high level of sugar content and is processed. The manufacturers even add artificial colors such as red 40 and red 3 dyes which is harmful to our health if consumed in excess.

Soy sauce: This condiment is known to be used in a lot of Asian inspired dishes. Even though it's low in calories and is a good source of vitamins and minerals such as riboflavin and vitamin B-6, one should note it's high sodium content. Too much sodium in the foods we eat can leave us feeling bloated and put us at a greater risk of developing hypertension. It is best to try the lighter versions of the sauce which will have less sodium even though this may only be a difference of 300 milligrams of sodium.

Chapter 2: water fasting

Fasting has been around for years, it is commonly used by people who engage in spiritual activities like pastor, priest and Muslim. Anybody can engage in fasting because it helps for the development of our mental, spiritual and physical well being.

One of the great way to fast is by the use of water. When you say water, it means fasting with water alone, you don't need other things to add to the fasting adding other things like tea and drink are not included, it involve fasting on water and water alone.

You may think fasting with only water is hard, it is not hard, and the thing is as you begin to do it your body begins to get use to it, fasting with water alone is great for people. Fasting is very good for weight loss and aging but the thing is before you engage in water fasting it is good for you to consult a doctor. If you are on medication, it is advisable not to engage in water fasting.

Chapter 3: benefits of autophagy

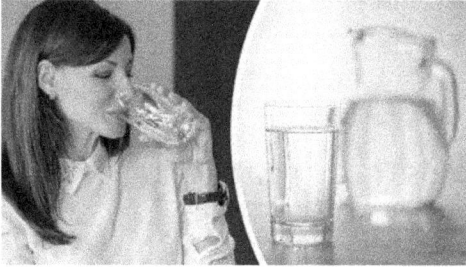

Let us talk about the health benefits in further length. Many people know there are numerous benefits to autophagy; the major ones are weight loss and cell rejuvenation. Even though these are great benefits, there are many more which autophagy provides you with.

In this chapter, we will talk about all the benefits that come along autophagy. There are many compelling benefits which you might not even know about, so we will go step by step thru each interest. If you are iffy about starting autophagy, then this chapter might turn you on to the idea of fasting. Without wasting any more time, let's talk about the positives of autophagy and how it can help you.

Weight-loss in a healthy manner

As you know, there are many ways to lose weight. However, one of the most popular methods being used to lose weight is autophagy, and there is a good reason behind it. Many people don't know this, but autophagy is perhaps the best way for someone to lose "body fat" instead of "bodyweight." When following most diets, followers tend to lose a ton of weight, but most of the time it is muscle and water weight they are losing.

On the other hand, autophagy makes you lose more body fat. Here is how it works, when you are autophagy for a prolonged period, you have burned out all your glycogen stores. Which makes the body hit your reserves, and that of course, is your body fat. You will be burning more body fat, instead of muscle mass or glycogen, which makes it ideal for people looking to lose weight. Also, as you know, autophagy plays a huge role in affecting your hormones. Your insulin will flat line, and your growth hormone will go up, this will prime your body to burn body fat instead and will do so in a healthy manner.

Now the main reason why autophagy works is pretty simple when you break your fast you have a tiny eating window. This allows you to stay in a caloric deficit, which makes you lose weight in the long run. Unless you binge eat, you will healthily lose weight. According to a 2014 study, people following autophagy lost a significant amount of body weight. Autophagy was found to reduce weight by 3-8% over 3-24 weeks. When examined even further, the participants lost 0.55 lbs. a week on average. However, participants who followed the alternative day autophagy lost 1.65 pounds a week, making it a much better-suited tool for people looking to lose weight.

Another way autophagy is healthier when compared to other weight-loss diets is the fact that there are no restrictions on foods. When people follow different diets it makes it very hard for them to follow since they have to eat every two hours and many other jargons, autophagy makes it very simple for you as there isn't a lot to think about. Where different diets make your weight loss goals your job, autophagy makes it super easy for you, and this makes autophagy a healthy and sustainable way to lose bodyweight. Overall, autophagy is a very healthy and sustainable way to lose body-fat. If you are looking to get rid of excess body fat, then you have nothing else to look for, autophagy is the answer for you. Besides weight loss, autophagy comes with other benefits, which we already talked about. However, now we will go into further details of the health benefits autophagy comes with when you start.

Increased longevity

There have been many studies showing that autophagy can boost longevity. As you might know by now that autophagy can help with cell rejuvenation or also known as autophagy, this process enables you to get rid of the old and weak cell and replace it with newer stronger ones. This process has shown to increase longevity and overall well-being, which is one of the reasons why autophagy can help you live a longer life. Moreover, some studies are showing that reducing calories in animals by 30% to 40% has shown to increase their lifespan. However, there is no study done on humans claiming such. Nonetheless, some studies are suggesting that monkeys that ate less lived longer. However, there was another study indicating that it wasn't the case on 25-year-old long research done by another party.

Although there is no actual study backing these claims up, it does show that people who ate less had a fewer risk of diseases which could lead to longevity. Which is excellent news when looking at it from that angle, there is a lot of disease prevention that comes with autophagy, but we will talk about those later in this chapter? However, the main thing to remember would be the fact that autophagy helps with autophagy, which enables you to rejuvenate cells, which makes it very evident that autophagy can help you with longevity and overall well-being, which is a great thing to consider.

Prevent diseases

There are many diseases present in today's day and age, and it very common to meet someone suffering from one. Which means, we need to figure out a way to reduce the risk of diseases for overall health and well-being? Intermittent has shown to lower risk of many diseases, and we will be discussing all the conditions autophagy can help getting rid. One of the many diseases autophagy could be Alzheimer's and Parkinson's.

As you know, autophagy helps with boost brain health and to lower the risk of neurogenic diseases. Some studies are showing that autophagy can help reduce the risk of depression, even though some people might not consider this a condition; it is still a significant issue in our society. Autophagy has also shown to reduce cholesterol, a 2010 study on overweight women found that autophagy improved hosts of health complications including cholesterol levels(LDL) and blood pressure which is also known as the silent killer.

Autophagy also helps with reducing type 2 diabetes, and there was one study done on men, which showed that autophagy helped them stop insulin treatment.

Although we don't recommend, you try this if you have type 2 diabetes that goes to show you the power of autophagy and insulin resistance.

Nonetheless, many studies are suggesting that autophagy can lower the risk of diabetes. Another devastating disease which autophagy helps getting rid of would be heart diseases. As you know, autophagy enables you to get rid of hypertension, which leads to heart issues. Once your blood pressure drops down, your heart will be working a lot more efficiently, allowing you a healthier life.

In regards to a healthier life, autophagy has also shown to reduce the risk of obesity. One study done on obese women suggested that autophagy reduced the risk of obesity in women, which makes sense as it helps you lose and manage body weight. One of the primary diseases which autophagy could help reduce the risk of is cancer, even though it hasn't been proven yet. Many scientists believe autophagy for a prolonged period could help you get rid of cancer.

These facts about autophagy show you how autophagy can help you get free of many diseases, and some have been backed up with detailed studies, whereas others are still being researched.

Nonetheless, you can't say that about other diets out there. Autophagy will help you to get rid of many things, and prevent you from further having any diseases. There is no better way of getting out of illness or problems without the use of modern medicine, and autophagy is so robust that it will also boost your immune system which will help you avoid small issues like the common flu. All in all, there are many rejuvenating properties which come along with autophagy so don't overlook it and keep all the positives in mind before you look at the negatives.

Reduce stress and inflammation

Autophagy has shown a significant reduction in inflammation. As you know, information causes a lot of many chronic diseases such as Alzheimer's, dementia, obesity, diabetes, and much more. Now, there are many ways that autophagy helps you get rid of inflammation. The first one being autophagy, as you know autophagy helps you with cell rejuvenation cleans up itself by eating out the old self and rejuvenating them with the newer stronger ones. If your body does not rejuvenate itself with more new cells, the older ones have stayed for an extended period of time can cause inflammation.

As you know, the average diet does not allow for cell rejuvenation to happen, and this is where autophagy comes in as it has been proven to help with the process of autophagy. Another way autophagy enables you to get rid of inflammation would be by producing ketones. When your autophagy your body uses up all the glycogen stores which makes it start using stored fat for fuel, and when fats are broken down for energy ketones are produced. One of the most popular ketones in your body will block a part of your immune system, which is responsible for inflammatory disorders. Another way autophagy helps you lower the risk of inflammation is by making you insulin sensitive, and when your body becomes insulin resistant, you will be holding much glucose in your bloodstream. More glucose in your blood will create inflammation and autophagy allows your body to get rid of all the glucose, which helps you reduce inflammation in your body.

Now that we've talked about many ways autophagy enables you to reduce inflammation, let's talk about how autophagy can help you get rid of stress. You see inflammation and stress go hand in hand. If you have high levels of inflammation, chances are your stress levels are going to be higher. Which means that if you lower your inflammation, you will reduce your stress levels, and as you know, autophagy helps with better brain function? Autophagy enables you to send better signals to your brain, which would equal a better functioning brain.

When your mind is functioning at its highest peak, your levels of stress dropdown, better brain function will also help you get rid of any stress you might be having, and having overall better health can help you reduce weight. Overall, all the health benefits you get from autophagy will help you get rid of your weight or at least lowly it. Which means, even if you are not facing pressure, autophagy will help you have a better functioning brain and also help you get rid of any mental fog or stress you might be dealing? What that in mind, always make sure you consult a physician if you are noticing much more stress than you can handle, as it can be something severe and not fixable by autophagy.

Body detox and cell cleaned

Detoxing your body is very important when it comes to living a long healthy life, many people detox their body thru juice cleanse or other methods out there when the truth is that they don't work. Time and time again, autophagy has shown to help detox your body in both the cellular level and digestive level, which means autophagy is a lot more superior when it comes to cleaning your body.

As you know, from cellular level autophagy detoxifies your body with the process of autophagy, what this process does it eat out the bad cells and replace it with healthier and much stronger cells. Through this process, you will notice benefits such as a stronger immune system, prevention of diseases, and insulin sensitivity. It has also shown to reduce the risk of cancer, which is a great thing to know. Overall, this is how autophagy detoxifies your body from a cellular level. Let's talk about how autophagy helps you detoxify from a digestive level standpoint.

People say that your gut is your second brain, and studies are showing how your stomach and mind are connected. Which means if your digestive system isn't functioning at its absolute peak, then chances are your brain won't either? It is essential to have a gut which is clean and working correctly, and intermittent helps a lot with this process.

It has been shown that autophagy can help you clean out your gut and intestines out of debris and junk. Sometimes, we must give your digestive system a break from eating all those foods regularly. Once you start your fast your body will begin to slowly get rid of all the toxins present in your gut, you see when you are eating all the time your body doesn't get a chance to clean itself.

Your body has to focus on digesting the food instead of cleaning out the toxins when you give your body a break from eating. It will start to clean out its gut. Which makes this process great for people who are fasting, when you have a high functioning gut, it will help you digest your food a lot better and also think better? The detoxifying body helps you tremendously with lowering the risk of diseases, which will help you live a longer life.

By now, you can see the pattern, and autophagy helps you from every single place to prevent diseases and many other complications. Which means there are more positives than negatives with autophagy, as we go along in this chapter, you will learn more benefits when it comes to autophagy? However, remember that these will only work unless you do; you have to follow autophagy the right way to see these benefits. With that being said, I hope you have learned a lot from this book as we are almost halfway through it! Now let's move on to another benefit.

Improved insulin sensitivity

As you know, autophagy helps you get more insulin sensitive, which allows you with many things. To understand it better, let me explain to you how insulin works. Every time you eat a meal, your insulin spikes up, then insulin is used to shuttle food either to muscle or your fat store.

When you have too much glycogen in your bloodstream, your body will send that energy to your fat stores. Whereas if you're insulin sensitive, your body will send the glycogen to muscle stores and will be used for energy. When you are insulin sensitive, you are more likely to use up all the glycogen from your food faster, and not requiring your glycogen to be converted into fats.

How autophagy helps with curing insulin resistance is by using up all the glycogen stores, making your body use up fat stores and when you eat food again, it will use up all the glycogen and shuttle it straight to the muscle mass to be used for energy instead of being stored into fat. That is how autophagy helps you become more insulin sensitive, the benefits of being insulin sensitive are many. Once you become insulin sensitive, you will notice more mental energy and less mental fog, and you will also see less fat being stored in your body which makes it ideal for people looking to lose fat and or gain muscle.

Being insulin sensitive will also help you gain more muscle since most of the energy will be sent out to your muscle stores. It will be used to build stronger muscles instead of storing it into fat. Being insulin sensitive is a must, as it will also help you get rid of possible diseases such as type 2 diabetes. All in all, autophagy helps you tremendously with insulin sensitively, which will overall help you live a healthier life.

Increased production of neurotrophic growth factor

Believe it or not, autophagy affects your brain in a significant way. It all happens from the help of brain-derived neurotrophic growth factor, also known as (BDNF), this helps promote neuroplasticity. Neuroplasticity is your brain's ability to migrate and shapeshift, and this helps our brain to produce new brain cells. Once you have an ample supply of BDNF, we can preserve older cells while producing new brain cells. Which means your brain will be healthy and will keep growing because of the new cells coming. Multiple studies are showing that autophagy to improve brain-derived neurotrophic growth factor, more specifically when it has to do with synapses; this is where your neurotransmitter travel cell to cell.

Autophagy has shown to promote this, and there was a study done where it showed autophagy in process for 12 to 16 hours has shown to increase levels of brain-derived neurotrophic growth factor by around 50-400%. Now we know that autophagy helps promote (BDNF), more explicitly, autophagy helps when it comes down to synapses. It improves what is known as synaptic plasticity, and this helps modulate our moods better. For instance, we can strengthen a synapse or weaken a synapse. This process enables you to be in the moment when you need to be happy or scared; this will help you modulate that accordingly.

In layman's term, this process helps us change our mood and be reactive at the moment. For example, if you need to be more focused, you will be able to because you are modulating it. When your brain-derived neurotrophic growth factor increases, so do your (BDNF) expression. This process helps you produce more brain cells and protect more brain cells, and this affects your cells at a genetic level altering our DNA. Which makes autophagy one of the best ways to protect your brain, and this gives your mind all the help it needs to preserve and recycle out old cells.

Another thing which it helps with is producing more growth hormone, and there was a study done where it showed upwards of a 4000% increase in growth hormone levels. Which is huge when it comes to improvements, as you know, growth hormone is responsible for many things of them being weight loss. It is a plus to have higher amounts of growth hormone, in both men and women. I know that the information was very scientific, so to put in straightforward terms, your brain will rejuvenate a lot quicker.

It will also help you with controlling your moods, which will make it easy to adapt at the moment. Brain-derived neurotrophic growth factor will also help you produce higher levels of growth hormone and serotonin, which are both crucial for mental well-being. Overall, this makes autophagy one of the best brain improving eating patterns out there. For readers looking for mental clarity and fewer moods swings throughout the day, autophagy is your answer to all.

Boost immune system

There is a reason why having a healthy immune system is fundamental, as it will help you get less sick and be more "immune" to disease. Autophagy has shown to increase the immune system, so we will talk about how it boosts the immune system. There was a study done on stem cells when it comes down to autophagy, more specifically, they took a look at how the stem cells rejuvenated.

The study concluded that autophagy depleted white blood cells, which is precisely what we want so our body can produce better and more efficient batteries, which lead to more production of stem cells and lesser of white cells. Once you start to get rid of your old white blood cells, you will begin to produce new ones which will overall help you recover faster. This study also found that there was a reduced amount of protein kinase A (PKA), which allows the stem cells to regenerate. If you have a lower amount of (PKA), this means that it will enable the cells to turn on the regeneration mode, which will allow them to create new cells.

As you know, autophagy has shown to reduce insulin levels, which is a great thing for someone looking to boost their immune system. There was a study done showing that high amounts of insulin levels, prevented t cells from doing its job effectively. The t cells are here to suppress inflammation and to fight off illness; t cells are most of the time responsible for getting rid of toxins which cause disease and inflammation. When your insulin levels are high, t cells are not performing at their highest potential, which creates our immune system to the dropdown.

When you are fasting, there isn't a requirement for insulin spikes, which lets our body help the t cells work at a higher level and overall boosting our immune system. Since you aren't eating for a long time, this will give your gut a break. When you eat a big meal, around 70% of the blood and energy goes to your stomach to digest it. Which means when you are autophagy you, give your body a chance to recover. Everything is healing when you are fasting, which includes the digestive system. Meaning, your gut will be working a lot more effectively once you have given it some time to heal.

As you know, digestion plays a massive role in both our mental health and immune system, about 60% of our immune system is in our colon, which means when you are autophagy, you are recovering your whole body and overall boosting your immune system. You will be doing yourself a tremendous service if you can manage to boost your immune system, and with all the backed up science showing how autophagy can help you promote your immune system and reduce many other health problems, there is no reason not to start autophagy as soon as possible.

More energy and muscle mass increased

Even if your goal isn't to put on more muscle, it is still good to have more muscle mass as it helps you with many things. However, the main thing having higher amounts of muscle mass helps you with would be a fat loss; having a higher muscle mass will help you burn fatter since it increases your metabolic rate. Don't worry and you don't have to look like a bodybuilder for that to happen; nonetheless, it is essential to have the right amount of muscle mass, especially for women.

Autophagy has shown to increase and preserve muscle mass, so let's talk about how that happens. There was a study done between two groups of me one followed a 16/8 autophagy method, and the others followed, whereas the other followed a regular eating pattern. Both groups followed the same workout and the same diet, and just the group autophagy would eat in the eight-hour window. What they noticed after eight weeks was, both the groups gained and preserved the same amount of muscle, but the group who were following the autophagy lost more fat.

This shows that autophagy not only helped followers gain muscle and preserve it, but it also helped them lose fat simultaneously. The main reason behind that is growth hormone, as you know; autophagy has shown to increase growth hormone in our bodies. What growth hormone mainly does, it allows a lot less muscle breakdown and to burn more fat, which is one of the main reasons why autophagy is so beneficial for building and preserving muscle mass.

Another great benefit of autophagy, as you know, is higher energy levels, and there is a reason behind it. Many people know how it feels to have a sugar crash, you feel tired and lethargic, and the culprit behind it is insulin. When insulin is spiked up, your energy level goes down as this gives your brain a signal to relax. When you are autophagy, there are no insulin spikes throughout the day, which provides you with more energy to stuff.

Another reason why you have more energy when you are in autophagy is that your body goes into a fight or flight response and since your body is in a normal starvation mode, it feels like for it to get food it needs to hunt. Which is when your body produces more adrenaline throughout the day, which gives you more energy as you go along? Just be aware, at the beginning of your autophagy journey, you might feel less energized.

The reason behind it is because your body is still getting used to these changes, but after a week or two, you should start to notice more energy. Use the power to get more work done at work and gym. In my opinion, and this is the most significant benefit which comes along with autophagy. More energy makes you feel a lot better when you are looking towards making it thru those long days.

These are all the main benefits which come along when you start fasting, and the benefits genuinely outweigh all the negatives autophagy might come with. These benefits can be life-changing to most people, lowering the risk of diseases and increasing longevity it's a fantastic thing to have. Autophagy provides you with that and then some, with that being said It is now time for you to pick an autophagy plan and start implementing it which is what we are going to talk about in the next chapter.

Chapter 4: autophagy and intermittent fasting

Do you know what the best thing about intermittent fasting is? Weight loss and better health are undoubtedly good reasons; however, the answer is autophagy. Do you know what autophagy is? Read on to learn more about autophagy and how intermittent fasting helps.

There are different reasons why people opt for intermittent fasting, and the reasons can range from weight loss to convenience. Restricting yourself to an eating window of just a couple of hours daily puts your body into a state of calorie deficit, but using intermittent fasting to lose weight is merely a partial benefit.

Juice cleanses and detox diets don't work. They are merely fad diets, and like all fads, they will fade away. There is nothing wrong with having a kale smoothie to flush the toxins out of your system; however, there is a better way to get rid of toxins. Our bodies can cleanse themselves, and it is via a process that you can fully control. All you need to do is trigger the self-cannibalism metabolism of your body. It might sound slightly scary, but it is quite natural and perfect for your overall health. Does that seem dubious? It isn't, and you can train your body to eat itself. It is known as autophagy, and it helps to cleanse your body. Apart from all the toxins in the body, there are plenty of dead and diseased cells as well.

In autophagy, your body gobbles up these cells and helps to make new ones in their place. You have to send your car for servicing from time to time, even if it functions well. You have to replace the oil in your car, and certain new parts have to be installed. In the same manner, your body needs to be serviced from time to time to make it more efficient. The faulty parts would need to be removed, and new ones put in their place. Well, autophagy does this for you.

Autophagocytosis is the technical term for autophagy. Autophagy might sound slightly scary, but it is an entirely natural process. It is a body mechanism that helps to disassemble our cells and get rid of all their components that are dysfunctional. It essentially means that your body is in a recycle mode and gets rid of all the waste that's accumulated within. Autophagy places your body in a catabolic state wherein it starts to break down its tissue instead of an anabolic state where it builds tissue.

There are plenty of benefits that autophagy offers. It helps to reduce inflammation in the body and strengthens your immune system. Autophagy also slows down the process of aging and suppresses the growth of cancerous cells and tumors. It also kills any infectious particles and toxins present in the body.

The lack of autophagy leads to weight gain, laziness, impairment of the brain and high levels of cholesterol.

So, how does autophagy work? When your body triggers autophagy, the cells present in your body hunt for all the dead or malfunctioning cells and destroys them. Destroy might not be the right word; the healthy cells devour the unhealthy cells. It involves the creation of a double membrane around a cell that's going to be eaten, and it is known as an autophagosome. The diseased cell or the toxic protein is dissolved by the autophagosome, and it produces energy. How does your body regulate autophagy? The main triggers of autophagy are two types of protein enzymes known as mTOR and AMPK. mTOR is responsible for the growth of cells and the synthesis of proteins as well as anabolism. It helps to activate the insulin receptors in the body and helps the body create new tissue. AMPK activates a protein kinase that helps to balance energy levels when energy levels in the body are depleted.

How does intermittent fasting support autophagy? Intermittent fasting helps to trigger autophagy due to caloric deficiency. The reduction in the calorie intake helps the healthy cells to get rid of unnecessary proteins and break these down to release amino acids that provide energy. Intermittent fasting helps to improve your overall health, and prolongs your lifespan as well. Autophagy is the main reason for the benefits that intermittent fasting provides. Autophagy kicks in due to calorie restriction. You might wonder if a diet that prescribes small meals with little calorie intake might have similar benefits; however, it doesn't work like that. If you continuously provide your body with nutrition, it cannot enter autophagy. Two conditions are essential to autophagy. The first condition is the reduction of calorie intake and the second condition is a period of fast. When you fast, your body reaches for its reserves to provide energy. If you continuously supply it fuel, it doesn't have to process any fats or process any additional proteins. Your body is better off without any calories while you fast, instead of breaking the fast with a couple of calories and efficiently stopping autophagy. It is a good idea to follow the protocols of intermittent fasting, if not daily, then at least a couple of times a week.

Imagine if you have three square meals daily. You stop eating at 8 p.m., and you fast throughout the night. The first morsel of food you consume will be at 8 a.m. the following day. There is a gap of 12 hours between your meals; however, your body needs anywhere between 6 to 8 hours to fully digest the food you eat before it can shift into a fasted state. In practice, your fast doesn't start until the middle of the night, and you fast for only 6 hours. That isn't much time for your body to start autophagy. When your body is in a fed state, autophagy is low because of insulin and mTOR. Only when the fuel in your body decreases, does autophagy start. There is no fixed time for when autophagy starts. It varies according to the tissues in the body. As a rule of thumb, autophagy starts only when your insulin and mTOR levels are low. It doesn't happen when your body glucose levels are high. Your body needs to be in a state of mild ketosis with low levels of liver glycogen for this process to start. It can take anywhere between 12 to 16 hours for autophagy to set in; however, the process amps up after a couple of days of fasting.

However, it doesn't mean that you must starve yourself and stop eating altogether. If you do this, then you run the risk of starving your body, and it will negatively affect all the other activities you perform. Fasting doesn't lead to the loss of muscle, due to an increase in growth hormones and the production of ketones in the body.

Autophagy is essential to maintain muscle mass.

Your body can enter into autophagy if you do the following.

Try to fast for a period of 14 to 16 hours daily to put your body in a fasted state. It will allow the depletion of glycogen reserves in your body and keep your body in a state of mild ketosis all day long. You must keep your insulin levels low in the blood. If you keep eating carbs or protein, then you will suppress autophagy; however, if you consume more fats, then you will contain the insulin response in your body and help to prolong the benefits of fasting. It might briefly stop autophagy, but it does put your body in ketosis. Ketosis helps to reduce inflammation and boosts the health of cells. Regardless of what you decide to do, don't binge on carbs. If you don't want to trigger the release of insulin and mTOR, then you must control your carb intake. Exercise also helps to stimulate autophagy in the body.

A little bit of self-destruction and stress are necessary to empower your body to function well. Self-destruction doesn't mean anything that puts you in mortal danger. It is a simple process that your body follows to cleanse and rid itself of additional proteins.

Chapter 5: how can you stimulate autophagy?

Autophagy is a natural process whereby the body eliminates defective components of cells that can cause disease, while apoptosis is the programmed death of damaged cells. It is possible to stimulate autophagy or even cell suicide, thanks to diet and sports.

As much as cleaning is fashionable at this time of the year, you should know that your body does not accumulate toxins, and you have nothing to clean with hunger diets, juices or syrups. But maybe there is something you can do to renew yourself: encourage your cells to commit suicide.

The cells of your body are born, die, and are replaced by new ones. Your skin cells are completely renewed every two weeks, your lungs every two months, your liver every five months, bones every ten years.

We are like one of those Japanese temples that collapse and build again annually.

This programmed death of your body's cells is called apoptosis. The cells know when they have to die, and this suicide triggers when they perceive stress, either internally because they are damaged, or externally caused by other cells. This eliminates precancerous or cancerous cells or those infected by viruses.

If the suicide rate is excessive, atrophies occur: there are healthy cells that do not replenish themselves to the same extent. On the contrary, if there is not enough apoptosis, the defective cells continue to reproduce, and the problems are even worse: ischemic, autoimmune diseases, and cancer.

On the other hand, cells can be repaired by removing defective parts. As in a functional kitchen, nothing is thrown here, and when the cell expels the components that do not serve it, they are reassimilated in a process called autophagy.

What factors affect apoptosis and autophagy?

When it is time for the cells to die, a process of self-destruction is triggered. Caspases are activated, enzymes that "dissolve" proteins. The cell shrinks, the DNA degrades and breaks down. The remains are eaten by macrophages, the blood cells responsible for cleaning.

The good thing about apoptosis is that it does not produce inflammation or toxins, unlike necrosis, which is what happens when there is something that kills the cells.

Every day 50,000 million cells in your body die from apoptosis and are replaced by new ones. It is a natural, necessary, and beneficial process, especially if we consider that cancer occurs when some defective cells stop committing suicide when it is their turn.

On the other hand, autophagy (or lack thereof) is one of the decisive factors in the development of Parkinson's or Huntington's diseases, and encouraging cells to stop eating themselves has neuroprotective effects. Usually, when there is damage or the cell is repaired with autophagy, or commits suicide by apoptosis. This can be a problem when a cancer cell uses autophagy to protect itself from chemotherapy or radiation therapy, instead of dying.

How to stimulate cell cleaning

There are three things you can do to induce the cells in your body to renew thanks to apoptosis and autophagy:

• Intermittent fasting

It seems quite logical that if you have damaged cells, by cutting off the power supply, they will be the first to commit suicide, and indeed it does. It has been found that intermittent fasting improves from obesity to arthritis and protects against cancer, all thanks to the fact that fasting increases the apoptosis of defective cells. There is no need to starve yourself: short fasts, of no more than 24 hours, already have these effects.

The exciting thing is that it is not necessary to make a complete fast; it is enough to fast on proteins. It has been seen in the laboratory that suppressing dietary proteins for a few hours induces the body to think that it is going hungry, which has anti-inflammatory effects.

- **Sport**

If you do not feel like fasting, a very effective way to drain these defective cells is to create a peak of stress (of the good), that is, short and intense exercise. It has been found that running lab mice increased the rate of autophagy and improved the ability to process glucose. This coincides with the previous observations that indicated that exercise is a way to prevent and treat diabetes and delay aging.

- Control carbohydrates

When carbohydrates are reduced in the diet (especially sugars and starch), the body is forced to use fat as fuel, both ingested through the diet and the one stored in adipose tissue.

Fat is transformed into ketone bodies, molecules that serve as fuel for the brain and heart, among other organs. This state is called ketosis, and it has been used successfully to treat epilepsy, diabetes, and cardiovascular disease. In addition to all this, ketone bodies increase the apoptosis of tumor cells and appear to have protective effects against cancer.

What is all this based on?

HOW QUICKLY DO DIFFERENT CELLS IN THE BODY REPLACE THEMSELVES?

Apoptosis by dietary factors: the suicide solution for delaying cancer growth

These emerging data suggest that some of these dietary agents especially those that humans could be persuaded to consume may be used in the prevention and treatment of cancer.

Diet-induced obesity alters signaling pathways and induces atrophy and apoptosis in skeletal muscle in a prediabetic rat model

We propose that dyslipidemia can be a mechanism for the activation of inflammatory / stress-activated signaling pathways in obesity and type II diabetes, It will lead to apoptosis and atrophy in skeletal muscle.

Surgical Stress Resistance Induced by Single Amino Acid Deprivation Requires Gcn2 in Mice

Dietary preconditioning for 6 to 14 days of total protein deprivation, or the elimination of the single essential amino acid tryptophan, protected against renal and hepatic ischemic injury, resulting in a reduction of inflammation and preserve organ function.

Short-term fasting induces profound neuronal autophagy

Our data lead us to speculate that sporadic fasting could represent a simple, safe and economical means to promote this potentially therapeutic neuronal response.

Fasting: Molecular Mechanisms and Clinical Applications

In addition, by protecting cells from DNA damage, suppressing cell growth and enhancing apoptosis of damaged cells, fasting could slow and/or prevent the formation and growth of cancers.

Exercise-induced BCL2 – regulated autophagy is required for muscle glucose homeostasis

In addition, in animal models, autophagy protects against diseases such as cancer, neurodegenerative disorders, infections, inflammatory diseases, aging, and insulin resistance4-6. Here we show that acute exercise induces autophagy in skeletal and cardiac muscle of fed mice.

Autophagy clearance of aggregate-prone proteins associated with neurodegeneration.

Autophagy is an important degradation pathway for aggregate-prone intracytosolic proteins that cause neurodegenerative disorders, such as Huntington's disease and Parkinson's disease forms. The ascending regulation of autophagy can be a manageable therapeutic intervention to eliminate these proteins that cause diseases.

The multiple roles of autophagy in cancer

During the development of the tumor and in cancer therapy, it has been reported that, paradoxically, autophagy has a role in promoting both cell survival and cell death. In addition, it has been reported that autophagy controls other processes relevant to the etiology of malignant diseases, such as oxidative stress, inflammation, and innate and acquired immunity.

Ketone supplementation decreases tumor cell viability and prolongs survival of mice with metastatic cancer

The administration of ketone bodies caused anticancer effects in vitro and in vivo regardless of glucose levels or caloric restriction.

Effect of dietary macronutrient composition on AMPK and SIRT1 expression and activity in human skeletal muscle.

Caloric restriction activates AMPK and SIRT-1 to increase ATP production from fat oxidation.

Chapter 6: how to activate autophagy

WE HAVE SEEN that autophagy is carefully regulated by the human body through a number of triggers. There are many of these, but some of the more common include changes in food intake, hypoxia (reduced oxygen), and exercise. But on a practical level, most readers are interested in learning how they can take this knowledge of molecular triggers of this process and transform it into practical changes that improve their own health. You may be surprised to learn that it is much simpler than you think.

Because autophagy is stimulated by changes in diet, namely nutrient deprivation, changing your diet in particular ways can be a very useful trigger to stimulating this process. As we have already seen, the benefits of this process include not only improved health and wellness, but weight loss. Because nutrient deprivation, in particular, stimulates autophagy, many people automatically think fasting is the only way to stimulate this process. In reality, fasting is a very useful way to stimulate autophagy, but it is not the only way. Eating foods that mimic starvation and fasting can also do the trick.

The best way to approach this subject is perhaps to summarize the three main ways that autophagy can be easily activated, all of which will be explored in this book. Here are the main tactics:

- Fasting

- Diet

- Exercise

It is important here to make a distinction between fasting and diet. By fasting, we are referring specifically to eating regimens that involve periods of not eating. Many readers may be familiar with the intermittent diet. Although there are different ways to do the intermittent diet, this diet generally involves eating during a certain window during the day and fasting the rest of the day. For example, you might have all your meals between 12 noon and 6 PM. The rest of the day you are not eating (or fasting).

This is different from a diet (or dietary changes) in which you are not changing when you eat, but what you eat. In reality, autophagy is essentially causing the body to believe that it is in a nutrient deprived or starved state when it really is not. This happens because the body recognizes certain types of nutrients as indicative of normal dietary consumption, while others it associates with being in a starved state.

Because autophagy plays an essential role in muscle homeostasis, exercise can also be used to stimulate this process reliably and effectively. A good exercise program can lead to increased strength and muscle growth, but believe it or not, exercise accomplishes this by a process of muscle breakdown. What happens is, as you exercise you stress your muscles, essentially inducing them to break down so that they can become stronger and more able to handle the load that they are being exposed to.

It all boils down to homeostasis, one of the key concepts in this book. Your body tries to maintain homeostasis by constantly responding to cues inside the body that stimulate it to undergo certain changes. Lifting heavy weight, for example, is stress that lets the body know that it needs to change muscle composition in order to be able to handle this stress. This may mean recycling proteins to allow the muscles to function from one moment to the next, but it also may mean breaking down muscle tissue to make it larger, stronger, and faster.

A homeostatic process similar to what happens in muscle occurs in bone. This example is presented merely to illustrate how the body is able to respond to stressors at a cellular level. Bone is made up of cells that are constantly breaking down and building up bone. Although it may seem inefficient to be continuously breaking down bone, something essential to human beings, the body actually does this so that it can remodel bone. By breaking down and building up bone, the human body can change the shape of the long bones to meet the body's needs. People who ride horses become bowlegged because the stress of the horses back upon the bones causes the leg bones to be remodeled to accommodate the shape of the horse's back. It is all simple homeostasis.

Like exercise, fasting is a critical way to stimulate autophagy. Indeed, it is so significant (and important to most readers) that it will be dealt with in its own chapter. We have already touched on the fact that fasting taps into how the body evolved to handle food: periods of fasting punctuated by periods of eating. By simulating this type of diet, you are triggering the body to handle foods in a way that it evolved to. Underlying this normal handling of food is autophagy.

Using Food to Activate Autophagy

Dieting has become a popular way to change one's body because it is so effective. Indeed, as concerns about health and wellness have become more important in our society, people have become bombarded with a number of different diets that purport to confer this benefit or that. Many diets do not have the evidence to back them up, but one diet that does is the Ketogenic diet. The Ketogenic diet will be discussed here because this is the diet that has been shown to be most effective at stimulating autophagy (leaving aside regimens that involve fasting).

Many readers may already be familiar with the Ketogenic diet. Some of you might even have tried it already. The Ketogenic diet involves consuming foods that are extremely low in carbohydrates, supplanting them with foods high in fat. There are different types of Keto (with some more extreme than others), but a typical Ketogenic diet involves obtaining about five percent of your calories from carbs and about seventy-five percent from fat. Many readers have an idea that carbohydrates are bad because excess carbs can be stored to fat, not to mention that high levels of sugar can lead to diabetes and other health problems.

In fact, the Ketogenic diet is concerned about triggering the body to release what are known as ketone bodies. Ketone bodies are produced from fatty acids that are broken down and they can be used by the body as fuel. Ketone bodies are produced during periods of starvation and stress, although there are always some ketone bodies being released from the liver and used as fuel even in normal circumstances (although in most people the concentration of these is very small).

The three ketone bodies are beta-hydroxybutyrate, acetoacetate, and acetone. The reason why you need to know about these is that research has suggested that the production of these bodies is associated with health benefits in otherwise healthy individuals. The Ketogenic diet was actually developed to treat people who suffered from epilepsy that was not responsive to medication. It was found that stimulating ketosis (the state of having ketone bodies in the blood) was able to control seizures in people who had difficulty controlling them with therapy.

The Ketogenic diet has also been used to treat Parkinson's disease, multiple sclerosis, certain types of nervous system cancers or traumatic injury, and Alzheimer's disease (just to name a few). The Ketogenic diet is controversial in people that do not suffer from a medical condition because of some of the risks associated with it. Although ketosis can clearly be beneficial, it is also true that ketosis is recognized by the body as a stressful state. This means that being in ketosis for a prolonged period can lead to things like increased calcium released into the bloodstream from bone, kidney stones, abnormal periods in women, and abnormal blood work.

The Ketogenic diet, however, has been used to cause trigger weight loss, which it does very effectively. Indeed, the Ketogenic diet along with the intermittent fasting diet is arguably among the two most successful diets at causing sustained weight loss if followed correctly. The Ketogenic diet causes weight loss so successfully because this state is associated with the body breaking down fat cells and transforming fatty acids into ketone. Because fat cells are being broken down so efficiently to produce ketones, weight loss in the form of fat mobilization can be very dramatic.

The Ketogenic diet should be attempted carefully. A doctor should be consulted before starting this diet, and people with medical conditions may opt to try a different diet instead. As already mentioned, ketosis that is prolonged can cause changes in the body that can lead to health problems. What the reader should take away from this discussion is that autophagy can be stimulated by food by consuming a diet that is high in fat and very low in carbohydrates (about 5% of total calories consumed).

As you have learned already, autophagy is involved here because the state of ketosis is associated with starvation by the body, which is a stressor that induces autophagy. This actually causes the body to mobilize more fat cells and thereby causing fat loss to be even more rapid and dramatic.

Fasting to Stimulate Autophagy

Fasting is so effective at stimulating autophagy that we have devoted an entire chapter to it. Like the other triggers for autophagy, fasting is essentially a trigger that induces autophagy. As you have seen, autophagy responds to triggers like these because one of the primary roles of this process overall is to keep the body in homeostasis. If one is starving (or the body believes that one is starving), it is essential for the body to respond by downregulating unessential processes and shifting to alternative nutrient sources.

The body is able to respond to fasting through a number of hormones and signaling molecules. The idea is that the body needs to be able to recognize very quickly that it is not obtaining the nutrient source that it was expecting and, as a result, to shift to a different nutrient source. In the case of fasting, the body shifts to fat stores as a source of energy. Indeed, this is one of the primary reasons why the body has stored the fat in the first place: because our ancestors would have naturally had periods when they were not eating and they would have needed a quick supply of nutrients.

By having periods in which you are fasting, you are essentially triggering the body to mobilize fat for energy rather than using the calories that you would normally be eating. Again, because Americans typically consume a diet high in carbohydrates, we are usually in a state of both using carbohydrates for energy and storing excess carbohydrates as fat. The fat that is stored is rarely mobilized because our nutrient needs are always being met by all the carbohydrates that we are eating.

In the next chapter, we will explore how fasting can be used to achieve your goals, not only in terms of weight loss but for fitness (for any readers that are fitness enthusiasts). The Intermittent fasting diet, in particular, has been shown to remove fat while maintaining muscle in men and women who utilize this diet effectively.

Chapter 7: water fasting and autophagy

Water fasting, even though it is a fast, differs from intermittent fasting. This is because water fasting involves staying away from food and drinks entirely for a given period, the duration of the fast. In other words, you only drink water to suppress hunger throughout the fast. Water fasting can range from 24 hours to 72 hours, depending on what you want. It is, however, not recommended that you exceed 72 hours.

Worthy of note is the fact that people should be careful before starting a water fast. The advice of an expert, such as a dietician or doctor, is vital before attempting a water fast. People fast for many reasons. Two of the most important reasons are to shed off excess fat and detoxify the body (autophagy).

As indicated above, when you fast, you go without food for hours or days depending on what you want. The intention is to induce autophagy.

Pregnant women, people with chronic kidney issues, as well as people with a history of eating disorders should not try water fasting. This is because of the intensity of the fast and the limitations it places on individuals. We recommend a maximum of 72 hours due to the side effects that could arise from fasting. If you would like to extend the fast, the advice of a doctor is non-negotiable. Besides, you can consider retreat centers that offer fasting programs where you are under the constant supervision of health practitioners where you can be easily supported.

Worthy of note is the fact that you should not stress your body too much while trying water fasting because of the side effects associated with it. You might not be able to escape dizziness and lightheadedness on the fast, especially if you're a first-timer.

All in all, make sure you avoid driving or operating heavy machinery while on a water fast. The next part explores the benefits and side effects of water fasting.

Water Fasting Pros

There are many reasons why people fast. It could be for religious or health reasons. If you are going to undergo a surgery in the hospital, for instance, you will have to stay away from food. This shows that there is something special about fasting and health. Fasting comes in many forms. Water fasting, unlike other types of fasting, is highly restrictive because you get zero calories and no food at all. You have to be determined and mentally prepared, as it is not going to come on a bed of roses. With that aside, many health benefits come with water fasting. This part of the book will shed light on these.

Cell Regeneration or Autophagy

Since the theme of this book is autophagy, I believe it is okay to start with autophagy as one of the health benefits of water fasting. Cellular regeneration is one of the main advantages of water fasting. Also known as autophagy, it is the natural ability of the body to get rid of dysfunctional cells. Water fasting forces the body to go into an induced state of autophagy. What happens is that the body will have to choose which cells are relevant and functioning, to keep them protected, and also ensure they get adequate nutrients, since nutrient intake is limited already.

At the same time, the body disposes of old cells that are no longer relevant in the body. It also creates new, durable, and healthy body cells as a replacement for the ones disposed of. The ability of the body to get rid of these damaged body cells and replace them with new, healthy ones improves the healing capacity of the body.

Slows Down Aging

You not only get to enjoy autophagy with water fasting. Many other tremendous health benefits come with water fasting, one of which is slowed down aging. When there is an excess supply of oxygen in the body, it triggers an abundance of free radicals, which results in cellular oxidation, which also causes premature aging.

When you go into water fasting, however, the body cells already damaged by free radicals get expelled. This makes way for new, young, and healthy body cells, which translates to looking and feeling young. Bear in mind that when you expel old body cells, you make the body stronger, with a renewed capacity to fight off disease, infections, and germs. Hence, it is more than just aesthetic as some may think. Besides, new body cells can communicate with each other better to keep the body healthy.

Weight Loss

Generally, it is expected that when you stay away from food for a given period, the body goes into ketosis. It is usually not until you eat the ketogenic diet that you get into ketosis. The body goes into ketosis because no more food is coming in; hence, it is forced to turn on its reserve – fats. It derives energy from fats stored in the body and breaks them down.

Thus dieting, as well as water fasting, can get you into ketosis, which leads to the burning of fat. You, however, need to know that ketosis makes the body draw needed energy from body fat. As a result of this, you have to be careful about the activities you do during water fasting due to the restricted calorie intake. Feeling lightheaded is common during water fasting partly thanks to ketosis.

Improved Insulin Receptivity

The pancreas creates a hormone called insulin, which helps keep the blood sugar level of the body in check. When you fast, the body gets better at controlling spikes in glucose levels. Not only that, but the body can also send these hormones to keep the blood sugar level from rising. Since the body becomes more sensitive to insulin, there is a lower risk of developing diabetes now or later in life.

Reduced Risk of Cancer and Heart Disease

There is evidence to support the fact that water fasting does help reduce the risk of cancer and heart disease. This is not surprising, as this benefit of water fasting is the offshoot of cell cleansing (autophagy) and reduced inflammation.

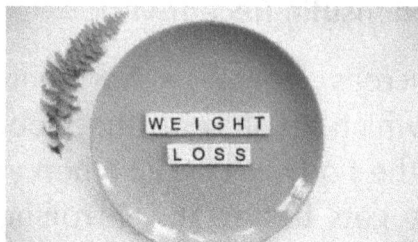

Also, there is evidence to support the fact that water fasting may slow or even completely stop the growth of tumors. Not only that, but it also improves the effectiveness of chemotherapy while helping to reduce the side effects. As a result, cancer treatment, when combined with water fasting, gives terrific results.

Also, as indicated above, water fasting helps get rid of free radicals in the body. This keeps the heart protected from any damage that might come from free radicals.

Reduced Blood Pressure

To reduce blood pressure, health practitioners advised limiting salt intake and increasing water intake. This is the basis of water fasting. Hence, it automatically helps manage and reduce blood pressure. Even people with hypertension can show significant improvement if they water fast under medical supervision.

Possible Side Effects of Water Fasting

As emphasized above, water fasting is highly restrictive. Hence, it does come with several side effects that you should note. This will help you decide if it is worth exploring or not. Also, it is essential I drive home the fact that the water fast is best and safer with the supervision of a medical practitioner. This is because they will be more equipped in helping to manage the associated side effects.

With the above in mind, expect and be prepared for the following when going on a water fast.

Dehydration

This is somewhat ironic; I must admit but bear in mind that the possibility of getting dehydrated is high while on a water fast. This is because the body gets some percentage of its water in the food ingested; however, water fasting restricts you from any form of food at all.

This is why dehydration is possible with water fasting as well. As a result, an increased amount of water intake is essential during a water fast. Keep in mind that with dehydration, the chances of feeling lightheaded and dizzy also increase.

Unintended Weight (Muscle) Loss

It is the loss of fat in the body that translates to weight loss. Although fat also serves as energy reserves in the body, it has no other use in excess amounts. One bad thing about water fast is that the body loses muscle weight, which is not good. This is because muscle is vital to keep the metabolism active even while resting, keeping the body from shock.

Muscle also helps as you go about your day to day activities. However, since the body has no access to calories while water fasting, you will not only lose shape fast but lose muscle weight as well.

Heartburn and Stomach Ulcers

The intake of food to the stomach is paused. This causes the digestive system to go on a break. Stomach acid with no purpose can trigger stomach ulcers and heartburn. The possibility of this is high, especially if you have had it in the past.

However, adequate water intake is a way to help reduce the impact of stomach ulcers and heartburn.

There are other side effects, but these are the basics. Bear in mind that one of the easiest ways to induce autophagy is via water fasting. It even proves faster than exercise or other means. This is why we thought to explore water fasting in detail.

Getting Started With Water Fasting

The best and safest way to go about water fasting is with the help of a doctor. Their expertise is significant in guiding you on what to expect and also to mitigate the associated side effects. Also, should any health conditions arise as a result of the fast, you will be able to manage with ease.

When fasting, planning is vital. If you have never fasted before, it is not recommended to jump into three days of water fasting. That is not ideal. As effective as water fasting is, if done improperly, it could cause more harm than good. This is why you have to plan well.

What to Expect During a Water Fast

The period of water fasting is a time to rest, not stress your body in any form. Since there is no calorie intake coming in, you should strive to preserve the little energy reserve your body uses to survive. Therefore, this is not the time to go out partying or exercising strenuously - instead, you need to sleep. Your body needs it. Be sure to listen to the demands of your body and give in to more sleep to compensate for the deprived energy. Sleep during the day and get 10 hours or more of sleep at night. This is nothing out of the ordinary. Embrace and enjoy the process.

Be sure to concentrate on taking in at least 2 liters of water per day. Of course, you are not drinking all this at once. Instead, you drink it throughout the day to keep yourself hydrated.

Water fasting comes with many health benefits; however, it will not come on a platter of gold, as the first couple of days will be tough. There will be unpleasant symptoms such as irritability, disorientation, and extreme hunger. The good news, however, is that you have a healthy body that can adapt fast. By the third day, you should feel much better.

When on water fast, it is essential you plan your schedule. We advise staying off work for the period of the fast. Or better still, schedule your fast for the weekend if time off will be impossible. Also, chose the fasting duration you want. If you are a beginner, we recommend a day or a maximum of three days.

Concentrate More on High-Quality Water

Fresh, clean, and high-quality water is the best to consume while on a water fast. Should the water you drink be laden with impurities, you will see the side effects quickly as the absence of food rapidly magnifies this. With the above in mind, be sure to concentrate only on distilled water while on your water fast. Filtered or boiled water is also a good idea.

It is important to reiterate that fasting is not for pregnant or lactating mothers. Nutritional deficiencies might hurt a developing child. Also, people with type 1 diabetes should not go for water fasting. People who are underweight as well should try other means to induce autophagy, rather than water fasting. If you have less than 20 pounds you want to lose and you want it to go fast, be sure you don't follow a protracted fast.

If you are determined and ready to go on with water fasting, make sure you proceed with caution and the right mindset.

Final Thoughts

We have introduced water fasting as one of the most efficient ways of inducing autophagy. Water fasting is an extreme form of fasting that comes with side effects, but tremendous health benefits. Water fasting will get you into autophagy faster than exercise and calorie restriction. However, water fasting needs to be regulated and controlled. Extended durations of fasting are best done under the supervision of a doctor.

Chapter 8: activating autophagy through exercise fasting keto intermittent water fasting

The autophagy process is like replacing parts in a car. Sometimes we need a new engine or battery for the car to work better. The same thing happens within each of our cells. During autophagy, old cellular debris is sent to specialized compartments within the cell called "lysosomes." Lysosomes contain enzymes that degrade old debris into smaller components for reuse by the cell.

Physical Exercise And Autophagy

Physical activity is interpreted as physical stress, but until recently, scientists had questioned whether exercise could impact cell autophagy and, if that were possible, whether it would result in any difference to our health. According to the study, autophagy affects metabolism and brings several benefits to the body, as well as physical activities. The work suggests that exercise and cellular cleansing are closely linked, but it is still difficult to define which paths they are going together.

To reach these conclusions, the researchers joined two groups of mice: One had an accurate cellular cleaning system, while the other had weakened waste disposal systems. Then the scientists put the guinea pigs to run along with a control group made up of normal mice. Shortly before that, the animals underwent a treatment so that the membranes involved in autophagy could glow in the dark. Thirty minutes after exercise, the mice significantly increased the number of prominent membranes in the body. This, according to the study, indicates an acceleration in the autophagy process.

In a second test, the researchers made a group of mice that were prevented from increasing cellular cleaning. When they were placed to run alongside the control group, those who were resistant to autophagy got tired quickly. Their muscles seemed unable to use blood sugar in the same way as the other group of guinea pigs. The biggest surprise came when scientists stuffed both groups of high-fat diets for several weeks until they developed rodent-type diabetes. The race subsequently reversed the health condition of normal mice even as they continued to receive the high-fat diet. But after running for weeks, mice resistant to autophagy remained diabetic. Their cholesterol levels were also higher than those of the other mice. Exercise has not made them healthier.

Regarding physical exercise, it has been observed that it can activate or inactivate the mTOR pathway depending on the area of the organism or the particular tissue in which it takes place: physical exercise turns on mTOR in the muscle and, however, turns it off in fat cells and liver cells

There are two other factors that can act on autophagy: vitamin D and melatonin. Both activate autophagy and this is an added benefit of sunbathing and sleeping well!

As you can see, there are different ways that are within your reach to activate autophagy: diet, fasting, physical activity, sleeping well and sunbathing are effective tools in the regulation of this precise system of purification and recycling.

Autophagy is a natural process of purification and recycling to clean everything that is no longer useful for our health and convert the valid fragments into new cellular components that our body can take advantage of in order to enhance our health and our well-being. The good news is that depending on the diet and the rest of our life habits we can promote this wonderful system of tuning to realize our full potential.

Fasting or Intermittent Fasting

fasting The key activator of autophagy is the deprivation of food. This process is closely correlated with changes in the levels of glucagon and insulin hormones. When insulin levels rise, the level of glucagon drops, and vice versa. When you eat a meal, the insulin level increases, while the glucagon level decreases. Meanwhile, when we fast, drops insulin levels, and glucagon increases. And this increase in glucagon levels stimulates the autophagy process. Therefore, the post is the largest known factor triggering autophagy. And it's not about limiting calories or any special diet. It's about fasting because even a small amount of food is enough to stop autophagy - glucose, insulin, and protein turn off the autophagy process, even a very small amount.

It is worth realizing that the post brings benefits not only because of the stimulation of autophagy. It also increases the secretion of growth hormone, which stimulates regeneration processes. But because to build something new we must first get rid of the old, the process of destruction (or autophagy) must precede the building process and it is equally important. We should also remember that the mechanism of autophagy allows the body to use all that is unnecessary, including viruses, bacteria, and other pathogenic pathogens.

Another method, less drastic, of causing autophagy is Intermittent Fasting, i.e. "Nutritional window". It is so much easier than fasting, for example, 18 hours, and during the other 6, we can eat meals. However, it is worth remembering that Intermittent Fasting combines with the caloric deficit so that we can be sure that during fasting the body actually reaches for "garbage", and not the glycogen stored in the liver.

Chapter 9: choosing the right fasting type

When you think of losing weight, then you have to prepare your mind and try to add more energy, look no further than fasting. When you lower your risks for ailments and enhance your memory, you will be able to have the fun of health benefits by having a change when you feed. There have been fasting diets that have been there for many decades, and nowadays, the trending fasting components are the paleo and keto. You will be able to get a fasting regimen that suits you, depending on how you feed and plan your health goals. Fasting fits into any diet, but you can enhance more structure because you have alternatives.

Never think fasting is all about religious determinations. There is a new phenomenon that is helping in weight loss known as the Intermittent Fasting (IF), and it is becoming popular in health and appropriateness trends. When using IF, you have to alternate amid the times you are eating and fasting. This can be referred to as patterns or cycles of fasting. You can use various types of ways to IF, but they will all come down to individual variance. You have to know what will work out the best for you when you have any intentions of trying the IF. For the first time, there may be trial and error. Many people have it easy to fast for 16 hours and curb meals to just 8 hours of the day. Some people, at the same time, will have hard times prefer to shorten their fasting window.

Are You Doing Well with Intermittent Fasting?

There has been a study showing the positive impacts of IF like weight loss, low blood pressure, and enhanced metabolic health, but still, there is a need for investigations about the long-term outcomes of IF. You can also look at the aspect of sustainability. When restricting or not feeding on calories for some time, it is not the same for everyone. Study as also shown that those using intermittent fasting rarely stick to it, unlike those using traditional diets to weight loss.

Even still, IF it has been the best effective form when it comes to weight loss. There are also other methods like feeding on a well-balanced diet alongside exercises. There is also another study that showed IF is not the best when it comes to weight loss or enhancing blood sugars. When you want to lose weight, then you should know that it is not a one size fit all tactic. IF is sustainable to specific groups of people, but others find this process not right for them. For you to try IF, then, you have to know how will you fix this feeding in your life, and this is when it comes to issues like social functions and trying to be active. There are some known IF methods, as explained below.

1. The Twice a Week Technique – 5:2

This kind of tactic to IF will assist you in covering your calories at 5oo for two days in a week. The remaining five days of the week, you will have to stick to a healthy diet as always. When on fasting occasions, then this tactic has an inclusion of 200-calorie meals and a 300-calorie meal. You must concentrate on foods with high fiber and protein to help you fill up and keep calories low as you are fasting. You are free to take any two fasting days as long as there is a day you are not fasting between them. And remember always to eat the same amount of food you feed on regular non-fasting days.

2. Alternate Fasting Days

This kind of variation has involved a modified fasting every single day. For example, you can control your calories on the days you are fasting to 500 or 25% of your regular consumption. Days when you are not fasting, you have to go back to your daily and healthy feeding habits. You can also encounter some strict variations that entail the consumption of 0 calories on substitute days as a replacement of 500. There is another study that shows people who follow this form of IF in a retro of six months has suggestively raised cholesterol levels after six months off the diet.

3. Restricted Time of Eating

When using this method, you to set fasting and eating windows. For instance, you can fast for 16 hours of your day, and you can feed for only eight hours of the day. Most of the time, people fast when they are sleeping, and this is a popular method. This can be operative because you will extend overnight fasting when you skip breakfast, and you are not eating until you get to lunchtime. There are popular ways like:

- 16/8 process: this is when you eat only between 11 a.m. and 7 p.m. or amid noon and 8 p.m.
- 14/10 method: this is when you only feed between 10 a.m. and 8 p.m.

This method you can try and repeat it as many times, or you can do it once or twice a week. This depends on your personal preference. When you get the right eating and fasting windows for this process, it can take you some days to find out, and this can work out when you are active, or you start your day hungry for breakfast. This kind of fasting is safe for a lot of people who have an interest in trying IF for the first time.

4. 24 Hours Fasting

This is a method that you have to fast fully for 24 hours. This will be done most of the time, once or twice a week. You can decide to fast from breakfast to breakfast or lunch at lunch. This kind of version of IF has some side effects that can be risky, like being tired, aches, irritation, hunger, and low energy. When you are following this process, then you have to return to a normal and healthy diet on the days you are not fasting.

Intermittent Fasting Isn't a Magic Pill

Whether you are using IF, keto, low carbohydrates, high protein, among others, they will all come down to the eminence of your calories and the amount you are incontrollable. What you have to know about IF is that; however, the jury is still out, and long-term effects are being investigated, you will be required to have a healthy and well-balanced diet when you are using IF. You are not able to lose or reduce weight when feeding on junk foods and excess calories on the days you are not fasting.

Side Effects and the Risks

This kind of fasting may not be safe for some people, such as pregnant women, children, or someone with some chronic illness. In cases that you have some feeding disorder, you are advised not to try any fasting diet. IF can increase the likelihood of binge feeding on other people due to limitations. If you are interested in trying the IF fasting, then you should be aware of some small side effects that will come along. IF can be partnered with touchiness, low or lack of energy, persistent hunger, sensitivity in temperature, and poor working and activity presentation.

Where to Begin?

You should put into consideration some simple form of IF when you are beginning. If you want to start IF, then its recommended to start with a moderate approach and restrict eating time. You should start by cutting out your nighttime feeding and snacking, and then you will go ahead to limit your daily food like eating from 8 a.m. to 6 p.m. when progressing and checking how you are feeling, you can decide to upsurge your fasting period. You should speak by a doctor or dietician before you begin using IF fasting. You have to take caution and go slow with it.

Intermittent fasting can be like the current buzzworthy health fad that will assist when it comes to losing weight, but professionals say it is not hype. A lot of professionals have recommended that the diet can help in boosting longevity and maintaining blood sugar levels and healthy weight. You can think that too fast is all about skipping meals and upping your intake of water. There are a lot of processes of IF fasting that can be used in any lifestyle. You can try to break down the kind of forms that can work or won't work.

1:1 Process the Least Sustainable Fasting Process

This is the least successful variation of fasting, which is known as the 1:1 method or alternative fasting. This kind of fasting is where you have regular feeding for 24 hours and then fast on the next. This can be applied once or twice a week. This process has been considered to be popular to kick start loss of weight; this can be least sustainable compared to all the fasting methods and in the long run, has been associated with eating a lot of food when you are not fasting.

16:8 Process of Fasting

This kind of approach will require you to eat for eight hours a day and then go ahead and fats for 16 hours a day. This is one of the most accessible forms of IF that you can maintain because you can feed daily, and there are a lot of meals that you can eat within eight hours. You can adjust the period to meet your lifestyle wants and characters.

Warrior nourishment will allow you to eat some fruits and vegetables when you are fasting. When you are on a warrior diet, you may tend to eat fruits, vegetables, and take liquids that have zero calories for 20 hours daily. When you are maintaining this kind of diet, you should be allowed to carry large amounts of food in the evening. This kind of diet will require you to have more focus on the quality of your diet, and this won't be sustainable to you most of the time.

Generally, IF is preferred to be the best for your gut. Intermittent fasting has been capable of increasing bacterial variety and has inclined the balance of valuable gut bacteria that can assist your body against obesity and increase of weight. Some people always think that intermittent fasting has several verdicts. Current research has shown that IF has diverse findings and won't appear to give compelling metabolic or weight loss advantages to the traditional calorie restraint.

IF it is complicated to maintain for an extended period, even though the method that you will take this kind of process will be hard to keep up with for a long time, this can be so to someone who likes to eat every time. When you have decided you will be using intermittent fasting, then you are supposed to consult with a dietitian. Fasting is not for everyone like pregnant women are not advised to practice this process. Some people also take their medication with food and such cases you will be required to adjust your feeding window to curb in your wants.

Don't feel discouraged, and try to move to a different kind of fasting procedure. The best thing you can do is to get your preferred method and stick to it, and you should not feel afraid to move to another protocol in cases where you find an original choice that you think won't match your lifestyle. The benefits are worth your efforts, and when you try and fail, then be sure there will result soon.

Health Benefits of Intermittent Fasting

When you are talking about weight loss, then you have to put some thoughts about why IF can work. When you first fast, there will be a reduction in the net calorie intake; thus, you will lose weight. Some of the benefits of intermittent fasting include:

Weight loss

Most people consider intermittent fasting with the aim of losing weight. In an article published by the JOURNAL OF THE ACADEMY OF NUTRITION AND DIETETICS in 2015, there are high chances that intermittent fasting contributes to weight loss. The study looked at data involving 13 studies and revealed that weight loss witnessed from the program ranged from 1.3% to 8% for a 2-weeks and 8-weeks trial.

It is clear that the amount of weight loss through intermittent fasting does not seem to be more than what one would expect in a calorie-restricted diet. Also, weight loss is dependent on the total calories one takes every day.

Reduced blood pressure

Intermittent fasting can help you lower your blood pressure. In a Nutrition and Healthy Aging study published in 2018, it was found that 16:8 fasting reduced the systolic blood pressure in 23 participants. Having healthy blood pressure is key to avoiding diseases like stroke, heart disease, and kidney disease.

Reduced inflammation

Studies involving animals have shown that both calorie restriction and intermittent fasting can help reduce the levels of inflammation. A study published by Nutrition Research involving 50 participants who fasted for Ramadan found that there were lower pro-inflammatory markers as well as low body weight, body fat, and blood pressure.

Lower cholesterol

In a 3-weeks long study published by the journal, Obesity, alternate-day fasting may help in lowering cholesterol levels and LDL cholesterol when done with endurance exercise. LDL cholesterol is known to be bad cholesterol which can increase the risk of stroke and other heart-related diseases. The Centers for Diseases Control and Prevention also noted that intermittent fasting can reduce the presence of triglycerides, fats that are found in the blood that can cause heart attack, heart diseases, and stroke.

Boosts brain function

What is good for the body is also healthy for the brain. When you do intermittent fasting, you will be able to improve your metabolic features, including reduced inflammation, reduced oxidative stress, and insulin resistance. Different studies in rats have shown that fasting increases the growth of nerve cells that benefits the brain. It also showed that intermittent fasting increased the levels of the brain hormone, brain-derived neurotrophic factor (BDNF), whose deficiency is implicated in depressive symptoms.

Protection against cancer

Studies have shown that intermittent fasting, particularly alternate-day fasting, can reduce the risk of cancer through the decrease in the development of lymphoma, slowing down the spread of cancer cells. A review study published by the AMERICAN JOURNAL OF CLINICAL NUTRITION also found that cancer benefits were observed in all animal studies conducted, which confirmed the benefits for humans.

People Who Should Not Try Intermittent Fasting

It is not advisable for everyone to try IF. This is because you can be in periods where you are not supposed to eat, yet you have some illness that can lead to a dangerous path to decline. The type of people who are not supposed to practice this method is pregnant women, those going medication on diabetes, someone on drugs, or someone with eating disorders.

You should be able to note that IF has side effects. You maybe feel cranky or hanger when you are fasting, and this may be due to low blood sugar levels that can interfere with your moods. You are advised to be on a healthy diet when you are not fasting. It can be tiring to make up for a calorie deficit if you have fasted for two days, but in the current society, you can access calorie-dense items that can be able to do it as suggested by professionals. You can maintain nutrient-packed choices like fruits, lean meats, vegetables, grains. For the first couple of weeks, you will have to deal with lower energy, inflating, and desires until when your body adapts to the process.

A lot of people will want to eat what the dietitian has told them. But with time, most people visit them to inquire about what not to eat. IF diet is the solution to weight loss, excellent metabolic health, and health and longer life. Before you start to give up on foods for some days to increase the process of weight loss, then you have to put this into consideration: the medical and nutritionist experts that have to advise you about fasting and weight loss. They will tell you about focusing on enhancing a balanced diet, then you will have to get the experience of starvation, and with so much care, you are allowed to try the practice.

Intermittent fasting has been considered to be a worldwide known health and fitness trend. A lot of people have opted to use it to reduce or lose weight; thus, this improves their health and simplifies their routines. IF has been suggested by a study that it has some powerful effects on your body and brain; therefore, this can make you have a longer life.

Chapter 10: autophagy's amazing effects on disease

Autophagy research did not only cover weight loss, but researchers found that this mechanism in the human body is so intelligent and is such an inherent part of our physiological functioning that it affects almost every aspect of the human body in terms of health. Researchers started conducting studies regarding specific health conditions and diseases that, in each of their degradative physiological processes, can hypothetically link to the healing process of autophagy. For example, scientists discovered the astounding effect that autophagy has on brain health. This means that studying a disease like Alzheimer's, which is characterized by cognitive and neural decline, can bring new answers if linked to autophagy studies. Some complicated research cases were identified at the beginning of this book along with the professors who conducted them. The fact that those researchers are already investigating and researching such a wide variety of ailments and the effect of autophagy on many parts of our physiology indicates a promising future for healthcare. We have, for such an incredibly long time, been told to take medication for different ailments and this has become the norm, based on research and successful trials. I'm not saying that we all need to throw our meds out of the window. There is a reason why a medical specialist prescribed them for you. However, self-healing or placing the body in a state where you enable it to create or support homeostasis without external help is ideal. It seems that, in our pursuit of health and longevity, we have moved our focus in some way to a more natural approach, maybe to discover mechanisms that can work in tandem with pharmaceutical medication. Before we go any further, it's also important to note that the incredible amount of knowledge that has been discovered recently shows that we still know very little about the human body, and when reading about all of the research discussed here, I think it may be a smart choice to keep in mind that this may not be the end of the story and that new research may still be uncovered. For all we know, this is the beginning. However, that does not in any shape or form suggest that we cannot start educating ourselves right now.

Autophagy's Healing Perks

When it comes to disease and medical issues, a weight-loss approach like intermittent fasting may not always be successful. One needs to consider the nature of each ailment, its symptoms, cause, and what needs to happen during the autophagy process in order to achieve improved health and effective results. These methods are definitely not as clear and well-researched as the ones that are tried and tested for weight loss and exercise alone, but research is in process and we can share what we currently know, which is definitely not discouraging. When we discussed the process of fasting and how the process is used to induce autophagy, it was clear that it can take quite a while—for some even longer than others. So, if you suffer from a specific condition, how long does your body need to be in an autophagic state to receive a satisfactory, therapeutic effect? Maybe there are other ways to induce autophagy for certain cases of illness. In the discussion which follows, there are unanswered questions, but there is also hope.

CHOLESTEROL

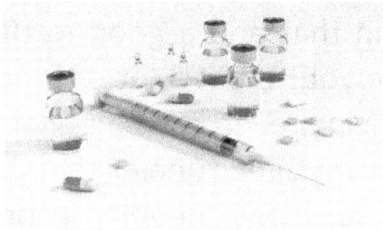

Most of us know someone who suffers from high cholesterol; it's like it's not even a big deal anymore. People's main objective is just to get through their day and get things done while not really focusing on their health. Could this be because our lifestyles are so terribly stressful, and putting food on the table is harder than it used to be? Not that anyone puts food on the table anymore. We all seem to devour it in front of our TV's without checking the calorie density or fat content. One of my favorite comedians says that, if you are even slightly close to being a normal human being, you will stumble into your home, grab the bread from the fridge and eat it by dipping it in anything runnier than bread. There's a lot of truth in that and a good Netflix drama can cause you to eat a lot of food without even noticing, even a whole loaf of bread dipped in anything runnier than bread. So, why do so many people ignore health advice and warnings about high cholesterol? Additionally, is there a way to lower cholesterol that will also address the causes, which are overeating, unhealthy eating, and unmanageable stress levels?

Well, if you decide to follow the 14/10, you can dip your bread in anything runnier than bread during your 10-hour feeding window. However, before you decide to do that straight away, let's look at what an expert, Dr. Jason Fung, says about autophagy and its effects on human cholesterol levels.

High cholesterol is a risk factor for heart disease that can be treated. The cardiovascular diseases that it's a risk factor for includes strokes and heart attacks, which can have serious and even fatal outcomes. High cholesterol levels are not necessarily due to a diet that is high in cholesterol, which has always been the main perception. This also then means that lowering cholesterol levels in one's diet will not necessarily be effective in lowering cholesterol levels in the body. This is because about 80% of the cholesterol in the human bloodstream comes from the liver. Another common belief that has been debunked is that following a diet low in fat will lower the cholesterol levels in the blood. This was actually proven in a study in the 1960s, but because the hypothesis and outcome of the research didn't agree with the majority scientific view at the time, the information was not widely published. The majority view at that time was that the amount of fat in a person's diet is directly correlated to cholesterol levels in the body. I guess it was a case of the minority being regarded as unsubstantial. This changed during the course of time as more studies indicated similar conclusions (Fung, 2016).

When we're talking cholesterol, and you want to get a clear picture of why fasting is effective in maintaining a healthy cholesterol level in the body, there are three friends I'd like you to meet. The first is my bestie and will be your bestie too, HDL. HDL or high-density lipoprotein is the "good cholesterol." Your HDL is a protective friend, so its levels should not be too low, as this can increase the risk of cardiovascular disease. This is why HDL is also known as a "marker of disease" (Fung, 2016).

Next, I want to introduce you to triglycerides. They are also a role-playing component in your cholesterol levels, but you don't want them to visit you in large numbers. In other words, you want low triglyceride levels in your body. An interesting fact about triglycerides is that they are also regarded as disease markers;

however, while an HDL imbalance can trigger disease, triglycerides can only be an indication (Fung, 2016).

Finally, I'll introduce you to your least favorable and more slippery friend called LDL or low-density lipoprotein. LDL represents your "bad" cholesterol and should be kept at a low level to maintain optimal health in the human body. Don't let LDL whisper sweet nothings in your ear; you know now that you need to keep this one in check. To make sure that you and LDL have a good understanding, practice regular fasting to show it who's boss (Fung, 2016).

DIABETES

Individuals with type 2 diabetes are not always overweight or obese. We usually associate this condition with being overweight or obese because it is also related to high cholesterol, a bad diet, a sedentary lifestyle, and heart problems.

However, let's change the perspective just a little by looking at how fasting combined with a specific eating plan helped type 2 diabetes patients who are not overweight. In other words, the focus was on treating the condition and not added weight loss (Hecht & Scher, 2020).

In this case, the patient was a woman with a BMI of 21.9 in her 50s. A healthy BMI for a woman can be anything between 19 and 25, so her weight would be considered pretty healthy. However, she has been suffering from type 2 diabetes for more than a decade and is unable to control the condition using normal measures that include a diabetic-friendly diet and prescribed medication. The patient had an extremely high blood sugar level of over 9% when she started with the new intermittent fasting plan. Just to provide some context, to be diagnosed with diabetes, your long-term blood sugar levels should be 6,4% or higher. This means that the patient's blood sugar level was up there (Hecht & Scher, 2020).

The patient started with an intervention plan that consisted of an intermittent fasting schedule combined with a ketogenic diet. After four months, her blood-sugar levels dropped to 6.4%, which is the diabetic marker. The prescription medication was then reintroduced and after continuing this routine for the next 14 months, the patient's blood-sugar level dropped below 6%. In this case, the combination of fasting and a ketogenic diet also didn't cause the patient to move under the health BMI levels, so she attained a massive overall health improvement (Hecht & Scher, 2020). If you are suffering from type 2 diabetes and you also need to lose some weight to fall within the healthy BMI range, intermittent fasting as a pathway to autophagy can be just as efficient. We've discussed how beneficial intermittent fasting is for weight loss and fitness, so if your condition requires you to make a lifestyle change, this is definitely a viable option. Always keep in mind that, if you suffer from an illness or health-related condition, the safest option is to discuss a lifestyle change with your physician.

There are also precautions that need to be taken when one decides to start a fasting regime to support type 2 diabetes. First, it is crucial to consult a physician before making any lifestyle changes when suffering from a condition like diabetes. Secondly, a diabetes patient should still give a lot of attention to their diet even if they are fasting. The fasting is not going to cancel out bad dietary choices, and combining the two may even exacerbate the condition. Finally, if you are diabetic and you want to practice fasting, make sure that you don't do extended fasts. Fasting for too long can have an adverse effect on your blood sugar levels if their regulation needs extra care and attention in the first place.

If you want to choose a safe but effective fasting regime, go for a 16/8. If you are not a diabetic, but suffer from insulin resistance, there are studies that indicate that the incorporation of exercise along with fasting can lead to the reversal of this pre-diabetic condition (Autophagy: The Process Changing Our Understanding of Diet and Disease, 2017). This is the cheapest and most effective way to improve your health and improve or even reverse the symptoms and effects of diabetes and insulin resistance.

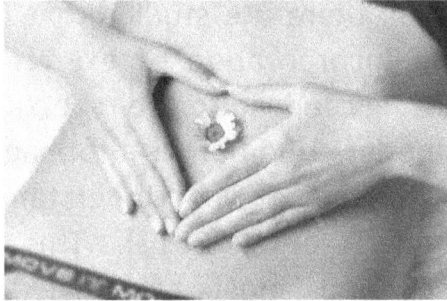

Autophagy can play a role in cancer prevention and cancer treatment. One of the most profound discoveries made by researchers is that, because autophagy promotes the death of cells, it can also be a preventive measure for cancer. This research that was published in the journal NATURE, goes on to say that autophagy can be described as a "tumor-suppressing pathway" because it acts like a checkpoint that prevents cells from dividing in an uncontrolled nature (Salk Institute, 2019).

The process starts with molecular tips on the end of chromosomes called telomeres that shorten each time a cell divides. The function of telomeres is to protect the end of chromosomes and to prevent them from becoming frazzled due to multiple cell-dividing processes. However, as the telomeres become shorter and shorter, and when they reach a point where they are almost completely gone, the cell enters a crisis situation. During this crisis situation, the unprotected chromosomes can likely fuse and subsequently become dysfunctional, and this is a trademark of some cancer types. What autophagy does in this situation is cause cell death, which means that these dysfunctional cells can no longer divide (Salk Institute, 2019).

To conduct a thorough study on the role of autophagy and cell death in crisis cells, the researchers also took an approach where they allowed cells to divide while observing the systematic shortening of the telomeres until the cells reached the crisis status. This time, autophagy was not used as a mechanism to stop the process by inducing cell death, so the cells kept on dividing and causing damage to the cellular DNA. This kind of damage is the same phenomenon one would observe in cancerous cells. The researchers concluded that autophagy's cannibalistic and reprocessing nature is an excellent way to protect cells from dividing themselves into a crisis situation (Salk Institute, 2019).

By subjecting the human body to autophagy, even if it is in a relatively healthy state, cell crises can be reduced or even prevented, which is a direct pathway to the development of cancerous cells. How incredibly awesome is that?

Alzheimer Disease

Alzheimer disease is known as the cause of advancing dementia that mostly affects the elderly. Alzheimer disease causes a patient to experience advancing, irreversible degenerative cognitive abilities. This neural degradation is caused by multiple pathophysiological processes, which include neuroinflammation, oxidative stress, mitochondrial dysfunction, excitotoxicity, and different types of stress, including proteolytic stress. The aforementioned processes all point to a complex degradation process occurring in the brain, which causes the symptoms of Alzheimer disease. Although extensive research has been conducted on Alzheimer disease, no cure has been found for this debilitating and ultimately fatal condition (Uddin et al., 2018).

Early studies conducted on mice showed that autophagy has the ability to slow down the process of cognitive decline that is associated with Alzheimer disease, and in this study, autophagy was activated in test subjects by applying methods of fasting. This was the first indication that the application of fasting with the aim to activate autophagy can lead to cognitive improvements in patients with Alzheimer disease. Up to this point, pharmaceutical drugs have been used to treat the symptoms of the disease, but no research has ever indicated a mechanism that can trigger a reverse effect or slow down the progression of the disease. Typical behavior associated with an Alzheimer's patient includes difficulty thinking complex and basic thoughts, changes in behavior, and the most common symptom of memory loss. These symptoms are directly related to the degradation of specific areas in the brain, where a dangerous build-up of proteins called plaques collects between nerve cells and proteins called tangles accumulate inside nerve cells. As these plaques and tangles start to spread, they kill vital brain cells the individual needs for optimal cognitive functioning, which causes the degeneration and subsequent disease. For many years, researchers were unable to come up with any indication or hypothesis linked to the cause of this degenerative activity in the brain, but more recent studies have led researchers to believe that it may possibly be linked to not only nutrition, but also the timing of meals (Jorgenson, 2019).

When calorie intake and Alzheimer disease was first linked and researched in tandem, experiments of intermittent fasting were also incorporated to test the effects of meal timing on the condition, development, and possible improvement of Alzheimer disease. This initial research indicated that incorporating fasting periods into the feeding schedules of rats indicated less toxic build-up in the brain and they subsequently had better cognitive function. They also lived longer. As ironic as it sounds, researchers speculate that, by providing your brain with what you would normally see as a starving period of fasting, you would actually be giving your brain the nourishment and maintenance it needs to stay sharp and young. This is because ketones that your body produces after using up its glycogen storage are linked to mental clarity, increased learning, and enhanced memory. Ketones provide the brain with the essential fuel it needs, and some researchers have claimed that ketones can provide the brain with more energy than glycogen. In other words, by constantly eating, we could possibly be starving our brains, and that is why it shows cognitive degeneration at a later stage in life (Jorgenson, 2019).

Currently, studies indicate that intermittent fasting is most likely beneficial for an individual who suffers from Alzheimer disease or has started showing symptoms. However, there is currently a new study being conducted on individuals who are not only Alzheimer patients, but also suffer from obesity and insulin resistance. This is to further investigate the relationship between not only food and Alzheimer disease, but eating habits and elapsed time between meals and how this can be a role-playing factor (Jorgenson, 2019). This most recent study is, at the very least, a strong indication that fasting is already established in these researchers' hypotheses as a role-playing factor when it comes to cognitive health. Consequently, it should also be considered a role-playing factor in the prevention and possible treatment of Alzheimer disease. If autophagy can help individuals to realize early on in their lives that they can minimize their risks of getting Alzheimer disease and be used as a therapeutic tool for those who unfortunately already have the disease, it can make a notable difference in the number of future Alzheimer patients and the declining life quality of current patients.

Heart Failure

There are many different types of heart diseases and dysfunctions one can be diagnosed with and it's frightening to think about. Also, it can happen suddenly with no indication that an individual had any serious health issues. Heart failure is characterized by the heart being unable to pump enough oxygen-rich blood to all the parts of the body. Currently, medical professionals state that there is no cure for heart failure and that more than five million people in the United States suffer from it (Felman, 2018).

Heart failure can occur due to a heart attack, systolic heart failure, or cardiac arrest. These three conditions sound like they can all be part of the same episode, but there are notable differences. A heart attack is characterized by a blockage in a coronary artery that causes damage to the heart muscle. This means that the heart muscle becomes starved of oxygen because blood cannot reach it. In the case of systolic failure, the heart is unable to pump blood to all parts of the body efficiently, so it is actually quite different from a heart attack even though it is also classified as heart failure. Lastly, cardiac arrest occurs when both circulation and the heart stop functioning, which ultimately means that the individual will have no pulse (Felman, 2018).

Some heart failure occurs due to a deteriorated state of autophagy in the body and the fact that it is not as effective as it used to be. The pathological progression that contributes to heart failure is due to the fact that mechanisms that are normally responsible for the reduction of protein are dysfunctional. This means that the maintenance of protein turnover needs to be regulated more strictly to prevent the risk of different forms of heart disease. So, where does autophagy come in? Macroautophagy and chaperone-mediated autophagy (CMA) both help with the transport and reduction or recycling of unwanted protein. The difference between macroautophagy and CMA is that macroautophagy takes big cargo loads while CMA takes smaller loads. Macroautophagy has been studied in research about the loss and gain of heart function, and both approaches indicated the significant role of macroautophagy from a pathological and physiological standpoint.

Fasting, Autophagy, and Mental Health

Mental health plays a pivotal role in our ability to conduct everyday tasks successfully and live a prosperous life. An individual's mental health can also be an indication of whether their physical health needs to be scrutinized and vice versa. Because autophagy can have such transformative effects in the brain and clean out all that neural junk that may cause ill health or cognitive dysfunction, why can't it be likely that this "cleaning-out" can also benefit conditions like depression and anxiety?

Anxiety and depression are sensitive to the stress we experience and whether this stress is acute or chronic. Acute stress is generally seen as healthy stress because the process is not prolonged and the body has the ability to deal with it without much fuss. It can even be used to improve overall health, as in the case of fasting. Chronic stress, however, occurs over an extended period of time and causes feelings of depression and anxiety. This is because the body cannot deal with a stress overload, which leads to negative symptoms. In both of these cases, the hormone cortisol is secreted. Cortisol is also known as the stress hormone and can be either beneficial or toxic, depending on how much of it is being secreted. In acute stress situations, less cortisol is secreted than in chronic stress conditions where a cortisol overload occurs. Unfortunately, chronic stress is more common than we think due to our hectic lifestyles and stressful jobs. The rat race causes our systems to pump out that stress hormone, so we need a way to counter and cope. Exercising is one way to cope with high cortisol levels as it induces autophagy, and by exercising regularly, you can reduce and improve chronic stress levels.

Depression has also been linked to inflammation in the body, and by using intermittent fasting to induce autophagy, it can have a therapeutic effect on inflammation, which can positively influence an individual's depressive state. A fact that is not commonly known regarding the subjects of depression and the treatment of depression is that there is a notable relationship between the brain and the gut. Good gut health is important for good mental health. This is where autophagy plays another pivotal role in reducing depression; it reduces inflammation in the gut by supporting the microbiome, also known as your gut's "ecosystem" (Rose, n.d.).

This interesting relationship between depression, your gut, and your brain is relevant to a balance of different organisms in the gut called dysbiosis, which can affect an individual's mental state, specifically when it comes to depression. If you are aware of such an imbalance, you can treat it effectively with probiotics combined with intermittent fasting. Then, you will know that your gut's sorted (Rose, n.d.).

Chapter 11: autophagy for muscle mass

Autophagy is just as useful for preserving muscle as it is at for losing weight. This is part of what makes autophagy-dependent programs a lifestyle rather than merely a diet. In stimulating autophagy through fasting, dieting, or exercise you create a new paradigm for your body that triggers a series of changes that leads to an entirely new health outlook. Men and women who experience fatigue, a weakened immune system, and obesity can suddenly find that they are losing weight, more energetic, and less prone to colds than they had formerly been. And all of this is due to finding ways of incorporating autophagy stimulation into their lives.

As you have already seen, activating autophagy is as simple as remembering three simple words: dieting, fasting, and exercise. We can also add a fourth word – food – but technically this is part of dieting. Food will be explored further in the next chapter as it is a simple and reliable way to stimulate autophagy. Dieting and food also allow you to improve your metabolism, which will not only lead you to look better and feel better but to have more energy and longevity. Some even describe a glow that people have because of autophagy. This is not pseudoscience. Autophagy has been shown to provide benefits to skin, hair, and other organs: all as a result of the improved functioning of the body that results from careful and considerate stimulation of this process.

Some of you may be wondering what autophagy can possibly have to do with working out and muscle mass. It has everything to do with it, to be honest. Autophagy improves your metabolism, increases your insulin sensitivity, and burns fat through direct lipolysis. These are all things that men and women interested in building muscle, or merely in looking better and losing weight, hope to achieve. Stimulation of autophagy pathways is essential to anyone looking to improve their bodies by adding muscle without having to resort to illicit performance-enhancing drugs.

Intermittent Fasting

This is a convenient juncture to begin the discussion of intermittent fasting, one of the most popular diets in the health and fitness industry right now. Indeed, intermittent fasting is popular even outside the fitness industry as many men and women have discovered how this diet can dramatically alter their bodies and their lives. Intermittent fasting has the term fasting in it, but it really out to be thought of as a type of diet. This is because, in intermittent fasting, one of the most important things that the dieter needs to do is to learn to pay attention to macronutrients as well as total caloric intake.

Indeed, it is a myth in both the Ketogenic diet and intermittent fasting that the total amount of calories consumed is unimportant. Although some people who consume high caloric diets as part of their sport – like professional athletes, bodybuilders, and powerlifters – might pay less attention their calories than others would this does not mean they are unimportant. In intermittent fasting, it is important to pay attention to the total number of calories consumed in a day and when you are consuming them as part of keeping track of your macronutrients (or macros) and in order to make sure that you are eating enough in order to meet your respective macro needs for the day.

In other words, in intermittent fasting, you have to pay attention to calories or risk finding yourself hungry because you did not properly estimate how much you need to eat during your eating window. This brings us to a discussion of what precisely intermittent fasting is and how it works. Intermittent fasting is essentially what it sounds like. It is a diet (or eating program) that involves a period of fasting separated by periods of eating. The duration of the fasting period can vary based on the specific regimen adopted by the dieter. Intermittent fasting is usually divided into two types:

- Alternate-day fasting
- Time-restricted eating

These are similar. They only differ in terms of whether the fasting lasts for an entire day or part of the day. In alternate-day fasting, the dieter spends an entire day (24 hours) without eating, while in time-restricted feeding the day is divided into periods of eating and fasting. Both alternate-day fasting and time-restricted feeding are popular ways of going about this diet with men and women finding ways of making the eating schedule work in their often hectic lives.

Time-restricted feeding, however, has received more attention from the health and fitness media because it has attracted a number of influential supporters in the community. This type of diet is popular for bodybuilders and fitness competitors who are looking to shed fat and preserve as much muscle as possible. Although calories are important and need to be planned carefully, this type of diet can allow you to consume high calories as long as they are within a certain window.

So how does the time-restricted feeding type of intermittent fasting diet work? It is pretty simple. The dieter comes up with a particular window in hours that they will be allowed to eat in the day and fasts for the rest of the day. A popular type is the so-called 16/8 split. This protocol involves consuming all of your meals in an 8-hour window and fasting for the remaining 16 hours. This would take the form of eating, say, between 11AM and 7PM (an 8-hour window) and fasting the rest of the day.

This split has been shown to be very effective at shedding fat, but you can use whatever window you choose. It can be a 20/4 window, in which you only eat for four hours in the day, or it can be more or less restrictive.

Intermittent fasting brings with it all of the benefits of autophagy that have been discussed in other areas of this book. It also has some benefits of its own. These have been elucidated by vigorous study both inside the fitness community and outside of it. The benefits of intermittent fasting are numerous. Here are some of them:

- Improved fat loss
- Improved cardiovascular functioning
- Improved glucose control
- Increased lifespan
- Reduced muscle loss
- Reduced hunger
- Improved metabolism
- Improved self-image and energy
- Reduced risk of cancer

- Reduced risk of neurodegenerative disease

Incorporating Intermittent Fasting into Your Workout Plan

If you have an active workout regimen (or an active life), it is important to choose a diet that works with your workout and other responsibilities. Fasting is difficult for many people because they feel they need the calories that come from food for their occupation, their workout regimen, or just for the energy to get them through a day filled with screaming children or obnoxious bosses and coworkers. There is nothing wrong with that. Intermittent fasting can allow you to have shorter periods of "fasting" in your day so you are able to eat as you need.

The key is to come up with a schedule that fits with your life. For example, if you need to be at work at 8AM and you typically go to the gym at 6AM, perhaps you should consider a 16/8 intermittent fasting split with an eating window between 7:30AM and 3:30PM. This will allow you to squeeze your eating period into your busy day. For those whose obligations are later in the day, you may want to push your eating window back a little so that you are not engaging in heavy activities on an empty stomach.

Little side notes about eating before a workout: many fitness enthusiasts have found advantages to working out on an empty stomach. Although your energy levels may be slightly reduced at first because you are used to having sugar constantly in your bloodstream, it has been shown that working out on an empty stomach increases your metabolism, improves insulin sensitivity, and provides a host of other benefits. Consider working out on an empty stomach if you work out first thing in the morning. You could always have your first meal in your window after your workout.

Other things to keep in mind here will be touched on in the Frequently Asked Questions section. Some are curious about what they should eat before a fast, after a fast, or whether it is safe for them to fast. These questions and many more will be answered. All you have to do is keep reading.

Chapter 12: autophagy and cancer

Cancer causes cells to divide without control. This can cause tumors, damage to the body's immune system and other complications.

Cancer is a vast term. It describes the disease that results when cellular alterations induce the uncontrolled growth and division of cells.

Some types of cancer cause rapid cell multiplication, while others cause the body cells to grow and divide at a slower rate.

Certain forms of cancer can cause tumors while others, such as leukemia, do not.

The body's cells are specific in action. They have fixed lifespans. Cell death is a natural and beneficial phenomenon called apoptosis (cells die and are then replaced - autophagy).

A cell receives an order (to die) so that the body can replace it with a newer cell that functions better. Cancerous cells do not follow this order (are out of control).

As a result, they build up in the body, using oxygen and nutrients that would usually nourish other body cells. Cancerous cells can cause tumors, impair the human immune system and induce changes that prevent the body from functioning normally.

Cancerous cells may appear in one area, then spread via the lymph nodes to another part of the body.

Causes

Certain conditions or factors increase a person's chances of developing cancer. They include:
- Smoking
- Heavy alcohol consumption
- Obesity
- Sedentary lifestyle
- Malnutrition

Other causes of cancer are not preventable. Currently, the most important risk factor is age.

Genetic factors can equally add to the chances of developing cancer.

A person's genetic code controls the division of cells. Alterations in these genes can lead to faulty instructions, and cancer can result.

Genes also influence the body's protein production. Proteins cany most of the instructions for cellular growth and division.

Some genes alter proteins that would usually repair damaged cells. This can lead to cancer. If a person has a relative with these genes, the chances of that person developing cancer are higher.

Some genetic alterations occur after birth, and factors such as smoking and sun exposure can increase the risk.

Other alterations that can result in cancer take place in the chemical signals that determine how the body deploys or "expresses" specific genes.

Finally, a person can inherit predisposition for a type of cancer. Medically, this is called hereditary cancer syndrome. Inherited genetic mutations contribute to the development of about 5-10 percent of cancer cases.

Types
- Bladder
- Colon and rectal
- Endometrial
- Kidney
- Leukemia
- Liver
- Melanoma
- Non-Hodgkin's lymphoma
- Pancreatic
- Thyroid

Other forms are less common. According to the National Cancer Institute, there are over a hundred types of cancer.

Effect of autophagy on cancer (fasting)

The component of autophagy that affects cancer the most is fasting. Fasting may help with cancer treatment. There is growing proof supporting the role of fasting in both cancer treatment and prevention.

Recent research has shown that fasting helps fight cancer by lowering insulin resistance and levels of inflammation. Fasting may also reverse the effects of chronic body conditions such as obesity and type 2 diabetes, which are both risk factors for cancer.

Also, researchers believe that fasting makes cancer cells more responsive to treatment (especially chemotherapy) while protecting other cells. Fasting may also boost the human immune system to help fight or prevent its spread.

Improving insulin sensitivity

Fasting may help improve the effectiveness of chemotherapy.

Insulin is a hormone that allows cells to extract glucose from the blood and generate energy.

When food is consumed in excess, the cells in the body become less sensitive to insulin. This insulin resistance means that the cells respond to insulin signals slowly and sometimes they don't respond at all. This causes increased levels of glucose in the blood and higher fat storage.

When the food supply is scarce, the human body tries to conserve energy.

It achieves this by making cell membranes more sensitive to insulin. Cells can metabolize insulin more efficiently, removing glucose from the blood.

Better insulin sensitivity makes it difficult for cancer cells to grow or develop.

Reversing the chronic conditions

Recent research has also shown that conditions such as obesity and type 2 diabetes are risk factors for cancer. Both are linked to a higher risk of cancer and lower survival rate.

Modern research has also illustrated the effect of short-term fasting on type 2 diabetes. The participants in the study fasted for 24 hours two to three times per week.

After 4 months of fasting, the participants had a 20 percent reduction in weight and a 12 percent reduction in waist size.

Also, the participants no longer required insulin treatment after 2 months of this fasting pattern.

Improving quality of life during chemotherapy

Fasting may help reduce chemotherapy related complications.

Recent studies show that fasting improves people's response to chemotherapy because it does the following:

- promotes regeneration of all the body cells,
- protects blood from some of the harmful effects of chemotherapy,
- lessens the impact of side effects, such as fatigue, nausea, headaches and cramps.

A 2018 study showed that fasting can improve the quality of life in people undergoing chemotherapy for breast or ovarian cancer. The study was based on a 60-hour fasting period (about 36 hours before the start of chemotherapy).

The results show that those who fasted during chemotherapy reported higher tolerance to chemotherapy, fewer chemotherapy related complications and higher energy levels when compared with those who did not fast.

Boosting the human immune system to fight cancer

Fasting produces cancer-fighting effects in stem cells. Stem cells are very important in the body for their regenerative abilities.

Fasting for 2-4 days protects stem cells from some of the negative effects of chemotherapy on the human immune system.

Fasting also causes stem cells in the human immune system to regenerate.

This study shows that fasting not only limits damage to cells, it also replenishes the body.

White blood cells help the body fight infection and destroy cells that may cause disease. When white blood cell levels usually drop during chemotherapy, it affects the human immune system negatively, and the body might not be able to prevent infections.

The number of white blood cells in the blood decreases during fasting. However, when the fasting cycle concludes and the body receives food, white blood cell levels increase significantly. They almost double in number.

Cancer causes cells to divide without control. It also prevents them from dying naturally, following their normal cycle.

Genetic factors and lifestyle choices, such as smoking, can contribute to the development of cancer. Several components affect the ways the DNA communicates with cells and directs their division and death.

Treatments are constantly improving. Examples of current treatments include chemotherapy, radiation therapy and surgery. Some people benefit from more modern treatments, such as stem cell transplantation and precision medicine. However, most of these treatments are harsh and largely ineffective. Fasting (one of the pillars of autophagy) has yielded amazing results in cancer patients. Researchers believe that autophagy is the long-term solution to cancer.

Short and prolonged fasting periods have yielded amazing results in cancer treatment and prevention.

Stay young forever through autophagy

Aging is the process of becoming older. The term refers to human beings, most animals and fungi, whereas for example bacteria, perennial plants and some simple animals are technically biologically immortal. In a different light, aging can refer to single cells within an organism which have stopped dividing (cellular senescence) or to the population of a species (population aging).

In animals, aging can be described as the accumulation of changes over a particular period of time. These could be physical, psychological or social changes. For example, body movement or responsiveness may slow with age, while knowledge of world events and wisdom may increase. Aging is one of the most important risk factors in human diseases: of the roughly 150,000 people who die each day across the world, about two-thirds die from age-related causes.

Aging is a complex process characterized by the progressive failure of maintenance and repair pathways critical for cellular preservation, which results in a gradual accumulation of unwanted macromolecules and organelles. The accumulation of such oxidized, misfolded, cross-linked or aggregated molecules has negative effects on cellular homeostasis and on tissue and organ integrity. The defective molecules can alter homeostasis directly by interfering with the activity of functional molecules and organelles, which can cause further dysfunction. This progressive decline in cellular homeostasis leads to aging, disease and ultimately, to death. Although our understanding of the biology[7] of aging has increased in recent times, the molecular events underlying this process have only recently begun to be explored. Interestingly, research in the last couple of decades focused on deciphering the molecular underpinnings of aging has shown that in many model organisms, the rate of aging can be controlled by altering conserved signaling pathways and processes, implying that the aging process itself may ultimately be receptive to therapeutic manipulation.

Dietary' restriction and aging (intermittent fasting)

Dietary restriction, defined as the restriction of nutrients while avoiding malnutrition, is the most effective way of reducing aging. Dietary restriction was first observed to delay aging and disease in lab rats about a century ago. Since then, the effects of dietary restriction on aging has been studied greatly. Dietary restriction has been observed to extend the lifespan of yeast, invertebrates, fish, dogs, hamsters, mice and apes. Different molecular mechanisms have been proposed to improve the positive effects of dietary restriction on longevity, including insulin/IGF-1 and TOR signaling.

However, it is currently unknown to what level lifespan extension resulting from dietary reduction is mediated by these nutrient-sensing pathways.

Aging (summary)

Aging results from the gradual decline in cellular repair and body mechanisms, which leads to an accumulation of unwanted cellular constituents and ultimately leads to the degeneration of tissues and organs. Decades of research have shown that the aging process is influenced by genetics and that many metabolic genes can influence aging by mechanisms still to be fully elucidated. Autophagy promotes cell maintenance by removing unwanted materials and by using recycled components as an alternative nutrient resource. This shows that autophagy aids longevity because an organism can recover more effectively from stress-induced cellular damage. Evidence that autophagy influences the aging process has been observed in different organisms, from yeast to multicellular organisms such as worms and flies.

Chapter 13: autophagy mistakes to avoid

Autophagy is incredibly beneficial for the overall health and wellness of our bodies. It's also an amazing anti-aging and weight loss force. Fasting, exercise, and good stress-management are the three ways to activate autophagy, but there are some common mistakes to avoid when making these lifestyle adjustments.

Not Fasting Long Enough

Typically, especially when first starting out, you have to fast for about three consecutive days before autophagy is activated. That being said, sometimes fasting for as little as 16 hours can activate autophagy, and it can certainly activate ketosis, especially if you have a high-fat low-carb diet. It's also important to note that the ketosis state itself is beneficial, and that's before autophagy even happens.

However, most of us don't follow nutrient rich, high-fat low-carb diets, especially when we first being fasting. That being said, if a three day (or longer) extended fast feels like too long, don't worry. Start slow. Begin your journey by benefiting from the rejuvenating effects of ketosis and know that once you work your way up to longer fasting periods, your body will be in a healthy state to trigger autophagy.

Putting Too Much Fat in Coffee during Fasting

It's okay to put a splash of milk or a milk alternative, like soy or a nut milk, into your coffee when you're fasting. However, a splash truly means a splash. If you consume more than 50 calories in one sitting, you'll accidentally break your fast and leave the ketosis state, which in turn stops autophagy. Even if you don't break your fast, a sudden caloric intake can stop autophagy, even if it doesn't bring you out of ketosis. If black coffee is too bitter for you, a milk alternative is definitely better than animal milk, as it has less caloric value and is much less likely to stop autophagy.

BCAAS

BCAAs, otherwise known as branched-chain amino acids, are a supplement sometimes taken by people who are afraid of losing muscle during fasting. However, this is not only unnecessary, it's counterproductive as well, since BCAAs stop autophagy and can even bring your body out of ketosis. The reality is that fasting done properly does not lead to muscle loss. In fact, because ketosis elevates your hormone levels, working out during fasting can actually help you to build muscle.

Consuming Artificial Sweeteners during Fasting

Even though they aren't technically sugar, artificial sweeteners will still disrupt ketosis because they raise the body's insulin levels and will subsequently disrupt ketosis. If you're not sure whether the juice or water you're considering has artificial sweeteners in it, don't buy it. If you want to add some flavor to your water, you can always infuse it with lemon juice or apple cider vinegar, both of which have zero caloric value and not enough natural sugars to boost your insulin.

Taking Supplements with Calories and Sugars during Fasting

Some people choose to take natural supplements while fasting, especially ones that enhance the autophagy process. However, some supplements have caloric value or added sugar, and consuming these during fasting can disrupt autophagy and even kick you out of ketosis. Vitamin D, turmeric, bebeerine, potassium chloride, magnesium, and reishi mushroom are all supplements that are okay to take during fasting. Magnesium supplements can actually be very helpful if you are prone to headaches, as headaches during fasting often indicate a magnesium deficiency. However, if you want to take nutrient supplements during a fast, it's best to stick to just one or two. Taking too many supplements can slowly but surely add up the caloric value to the point where it disrupts autophagy.

Not Getting Enough Sleep during Fasting

Most often, autophagy happens while we are asleep. Therefore, the quality of sleep you get while fasting is incredibly important to autophagy activation. Disruptions in your sleep cycle can stop autophagy from happening. Large quantities of growth hormone released into the body during ketosis, but this, too, can be disrupted by poor quality of sleep.

Never Engaging in Extended Fasting

Again, autophagy typically is not activated until about three days into a fast. If you want to gain significant periods of autophagic activation, then you are eventually going to have to work your way up to an extended fast. However, a 5-day fast once a month, or even once every two months, can help you to gain a great deal from autophagy in a manageable routine.

Fasting Too Much

If you fast too long, too often, or too severely, then instead of activating an artificial starvation state to trigger autophagy, you'll actually start to starve yourself. Though fasting and autophagy come with wonderful restorative benefits, you can't stop eating. You still need to feed yourself with healthy nutrients in order to survive. How much is too much really depends on your body. In general, people with more body fat can fast longer than people with low body fat. If you find yourself feeling weak, fatigued, or dizzy during fasts when you didn't feel that way before, it's a sign that you're fasting too much and not eating enough.

Not Eating Well During the "Fed" State

Eating is just as important for autophagy as fasting. Not only do some foods trigger or boost autophagic processes, but your body has to work that much harder to heal and restore during a fast if you aren't putting the proper nutrients into it while you're eating. If you go back to eating carbs and junk food during the "fed" state, you'll undo much of the progress that was made while you were fasting.

Not Exercising Enough

Exercising is incredibly beneficial during fasting. It increases the rate at which your body burns fat and adds more "stress" to the body to trigger autophagy. Since ketosis releases hormones into the body, you'll probably build muscle if you exercise while fasting as well. However, not everyone likes exercising while fasting, and if you have chronically low blood sugar levels, it may not be safe for you to exercise while fasting. However, if you choose not to exercise while fasting, then you should make exercise a regular part of your routine while you are eating. Living a sedentary lifestyle won't give your body the opportunity to fully use the restorative benefits of autophagy and can slow down the healing process.

Chapter 14: different ways to do intermittent fasting

Intermittent fasting is a blanket term for a lot of fasting methods today. That having said, you should expect that there will be different ways to do intermittent fasting nowadays.

It is no secret that it has become quite a trend nowadays. Some people swear by it saying that intermittent fasting has helped them lose weight. Some credit their extended lifespan to this mode of fasting and others give testimonies as to how intermittent fasting has helped them become healthier.

It shouldn't come as a surprise that different ways to do intermittent fasting have sprung up. Note that there are no hard and fast rules as to how one should do it. However, you should choose the best one that would suit your needs. Not every mode of intermittent fasting will be effective for you. The goal is to make it as effortless as possible.

In this chapter we will go over the common methods to do intermittent fasting. We will discuss each in detail in a later chapter.

The 16/8 Method

The 16/8 method or 16:8 method means that you will fast for 16 hours each day and eat only within an 8 hour window. There are no exact figures but generally you will be expected to fast anywhere from 14 to 16 hours and restrict your eating time to 8 to 10 hours only.

This method of intermittent fasting is known as the Leangains protocol and it was made popular by Martin Berkhan. This is perhaps one of the simplest ways to do intermittent fasting. You can actually get this type of fasting done by just not eating anything after dinner and then follow that up by skipping breakfast.

185

Let's say you have dinners at 8 you should make sure that you don't have any post dinner evening meals or midnight snacks after that. When you wake up in the morning you should skip breakfast. Let's say you had your dinner at 7 pm and finished it at 8 pm at 8 pm you should refrain from eating anything at all.

The next thing you will eat is lunch the following day. You will skip breakfast, yes. And technically you have already fasted for a total of 16 hours if you do it that way. That is the program for the men. It is recommended that women have a slightly shorter fast, which should be about 14 to 15 hours.

Now this fasting isn't called a dry fast. A dry fast is where you avoid both food and water. That means you don't eat and you also don't drink. Experts say that 24 hours of dry fasting is the equivalent of 3 days of water fasting. Of course dry fasting is going to be a very difficult practice especially if you haven't done any form of fasting.

You can drink water when you go on an intermittent fast. You can also drink some coffee or tea while you fast. This can help reduce the hunger pangs that you feel. However, do take note that you can't take in any alcoholic beverages during your fast.

On top of that during your eating window you are supposed to eat a balanced diet. If you're still eating fast food during the hours when you're supposed to eat then don't expect to see any good results.

Some people do low carb diets in conjunction with the 16:8 intermittent fasting schedule. Whenever you feel hungry during your fasting window then drink water or tea.

The 5:2 Method

The 5:2 Method is also known as the 5:2 Diet and also the Fast Diet. This method of intermittent fasting was popularized by Michael Mosley, a doctor and British journalist. This is another simple strategy where you eat regular meals 5 days a week and then in 2 selected days you will restrict your calorie intake to 500 to 600 calories.

Men are recommended to take in only up to 600 calories during the 2 fasting days. Women on the other hand are supposed to take only 500 calories during those days.

So let's say you want to go fasting on Tuesdays and Fridays. On those two days you will count your calories eating only 250 calories per meal for the ladies and 300 calories for the men.

Critics of this dietary method say that there are no studies that support its effectiveness but we have plenty of people who swear by it. Some don't even consider it as a form of intermittent fasting.

Eat Stop Eat Method

The eat stop eat method will require a full 24 hours to complete. You will also be required to fast two days in a week. This mode of fasting was popularized by Brad Pilon, a fitness expert.

So, how do you do the eat stop eat fasting method? Here's how—let's say you finished dinner on Tuesday and you want to start fasting. You will begin your fast after dinner on Tuesday night. The following day you will not eat breakfast and you will skip lunch. Your next meal will be on Wednesday evening—dinner time.

So, essentially this is a dinner to dinner fast. Note that this is not a kind of dry fasting. You can have water, coffee, tea, and other non-alcoholic drinks during your fasting days. The only restriction is that you should not eat any solid foods.

People use this type of fasting to lose weight. It is also important that you should eat a healthy and balanced diet during non-fasting days. You are not supposed to eat like it's your last meal during the dinner before your fast begins.

That will just defeat the purpose of your fast. You are also not supposed to eat more food during your non-fasting days. It would be as if you are stock piling food for the upcoming fast.

Of course this type of fasting isn't the easiest one to try and it is not recommended for beginners. Note that the drop-out rate for this type of fasting is pretty high and many people will find it very difficult at first. The last few hours before you can eat again will be the most challenging because people usually become ravenously hungry since they are expecting a meal in a few hours.

You don't have to go dinner to dinner if that is not the best option for you. You can do the eat stop eat fasting going breakfast to breakfast or lunch to lunch. You can follow whatever fasting schedule that works for you. Note that this is a challenging fasting method and some people tend to just eat their next meal after the fast rather early.

Alternate Day Method

Now, if you think that the eat stop eat method is tough the alternate day fasting method is even tougher. Again, this is also another mode of fasting that is not recommended for beginners.

Using this method you will be fasting every other day. Note that you will be doing a full 24 hour fast on fasting days. However, there are also other versions of this fast where you will be allowed to take in around 500 calories during your fasting days. Again that will be 250 calories for women and 300 calories for men for 2 meals.

Note that there are studies on intermittent fasting that have test subjects use this fasting method (or some version of it). The results of course vary for each version. Now this fasting method is not suitable for the long term. No one can keep up with this fasting schedule without feeling miserable. It's a great option if you are looking for healing and rejuvenation but it isn't sustainable. You can have a fasting week once each month but you are already asking too much if you want to do it every single week.

Spontaneous Meal Skipping

This type of intermittent fasting calls for you to skip meals whenever it is convenient. Unlike the other methods for intermittent fasting, this type of fasting doesn't have any structure to it.

In other words you are just skipping meals from time to time. You can just go on fasting when you don't feel hungry come dinner, lunch, or breakfast. You can also just opt to go fasting if you're too busy to cook or you still have a lot of things to do and you don't really feel hungry. Again, in short, you go fasting when it is convenient for you.

You will be surprised that the human body is more than well equipped to skip one random meal any day. You may be traveling and you can't find any food that you like then you can go on a fast until you can find a suitable meal.

You can skip 1 meal or 2 it's up to you and that can still be considered as a spontaneous meal skip fast. That of course falls into the category of intermittent fasting. The only restriction here with this strategy is that you should eat a regular amount for each meal and that you should eat healthy food with each meal.

The Warrior Diet

The Warrior Diet is another popular diet and it was made famous by Ori Hofmekler, a fitness expert. This is a 24 hour fast—

well almost since you will have a 4 hour eating window.

In the Warrior Diet you will be eating small meals consisting of raw veggies and fruits. Come night time you will have a feast. You can eat all you can within that 4 hour window at night.

This was one of the popularized diets to incorporate a form of intermittent fasting. Note that this diet also encourages a diet that is similar to the Paleo Diet. That means you can only eat unprocessed foods. The only food allowed is from natural sources.

Note that there are a few common denominators to all of these intermittent fasting methods. One of them is eating regular healthy meals. Another one is that you should shift from an eating phase and a non-eating phase which is why intermittent fasting is a great way to induce autophagy.

Conclusion

The detox world is a wild west of misinformation and mistruths. Too many people are trying to sell you something, regardless of whether it works and whether you need it. Pseudoscience and intuition also corrupt and overpower meaningful findings.

However, behind all the false information, it appears that there are numerous benefits to detoxing and practical ways to achieve these benefits. Through autophagy, you can encourage your body to detox itself and this can be stimulated through exercise, eating certain foods and fasting. You can also help detox yourself by avoiding exposure to toxins, making healthy changes, favouring organic foods and more. I hope this guide has helped you regain control over your health and well-being. Happy detoxing!

CPSIA information can be obtained
at www.ICGtesting.com
Printed in the USA
BVHW071540270321
603572BV00005B/809

9 781989 744963